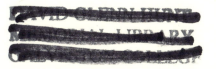

THE COMPLETE GUIDE TO
PREVENTING CANCER

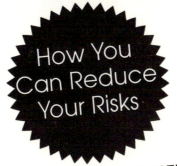

How You
Can Reduce
Your Risks

UPDATED AND REVISED
EDITION

ELIZABETH WHELAN, SC.D

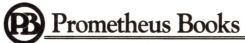

Prometheus Books

59 John Glenn Drive
Amherst, NewYork 14228-2197

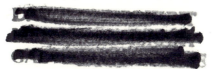

Published 1994 by Prometheus Books

98 97 96 95 94   5 4 3 2 1

Library of Congress Cataloging-in-Publication Data

Whelan, Elizabeth M.
    The complete guide to preventing cancer : what you can do to reduce your risk / Elizabeth M. Whelan.
        p.   cm.
    Includes bibliographical references.
    ISBN 0-87975-890-2
    1. Cancer—Prevention. 2. Cancer—Popular works. I. Title.
RC268.W528   1994
616.99′4052—dc20   94-11606
                                                                CIP

Printed in the United States of America on acid-free paper.

Contents

Acknowledgments

A significant number of individuals offered their time and expertise to the preparation of one or more editions of this book.

A very special thanks to Kris Napier, M.P.H., R.D., Research Associate at the American Council on Science and Health, for her tireless efforts in the updating of the original version of this book.

Also thanks to Debra A. Mayer, Research Associate in Epidemiology at the American Council on Science and Health.

I also extend particular thanks to those who assisted me in the mid 1970s when the first edition of this work was researched and written. These individuals (the titles used here are titles in effect in the mid 1970s) included members of the National Cancer Institute such as Dr. W. Gary Flamm, Assistant Director of the Division of Cancer Cause and Prevention; Dr. Marvin A. Schneiderman, Associate Director for Field Studies and Statistics; Division of Cancer Cause and Prevention; Dr. Joseph F. Fraumeni and Dr. Robert Hoover of the Environmental Epidemiology Branch; and many representatives of the American Cancer Institute, including Dr. E. Cuyler Hammond, Vice President (Epidemiology and Statistics); Dr. G. Congdon Wood, Director of Society's Section on Unproven Methods of Cancer Management; and Edwin Silverberg, Project Statistician.

Additionally, I benefited from the comments of Dr. Fredrick J. Stare, Professor of Nutrition Emeritus at the Harvard School of Public Health; Dr. Philip Cole, Associate Professor of Epidemiology, Harvard School of Public Health; Dr. Ernst L. Wynder (President), Dr. Bandaru S. Reddy, Penny Ashwanden, and Angelica T. Cantlon, American Health Foundation; Dr. John Zapp and Leavitt S. White, E. I. Du Pont de Nemours and Company; Robert B. Downey and Dr. Maurice Johnson, B. F. Goodrich; Dr. Richard W. McBurney, Diamond Shamrock Corporation; Dr. Vernon Riley, Pacific Northwest Research Foundation in Seattle; Dr. Albert C. Kolbye, Associate Director for Sciences, Bureau of Foods, Food and Drug Administration; Dr. David Schottenfeld, Director of Epidemiology, Memorial Sloan Kettering Cancer Center; Dr. William Nicholson, Mount Sinai Environmental Sciences Department; Dr. Farrington Daniels, Jr., Professor of Medicine and Head of the Dermatology Division, New York Hospital–Cornell Medical Center; Dr. Charles Black, Executive Vice President, Council for Agricultural Sciences and Technology; Dr. Thomas H. Jukes, Professor of Medical Physics, University of California at Berkeley; Dr. Judith Goldberg, Mount Sinai School of Medicine; Dr. Paula H. Kanarek, Assistant Professor of Statistics, Oregon State University at Corvallis; Dr. Perry Robins, Associate Professor of Clinical Dermatology, New York University Medical Center; Dr. William D. Bloomer, Assistant Professor of Radiation Therapy, Harvard Medical School; Jerome Heckman, Dr. Daniel S. Dixler, Dr. Wilhelm C. Hueper, and Robert Ferrante.

This work is based on the analysis of several hundred medical and scientific documents, but three publications were especially useful in my research: *Persons at High Risk of Cancer: An Approach to Etiology and Control,* edited by Dr. Joseph F. Fraumeni, published by the Academic Press; *Cancer Epidemiology and Prevention,* edited by Dr. David Schottenfeld, published by Charles C. Thomas; and the proceedings of the Symposium on Nutrition in the Causation of Cancer, published in the November 1975 issue of *Cancer Research.* Additionally, the papers and discussions presented in the "Origins of Human Cancer" meeting (September 7–14, 1976), arranged jointly by the Cold Spring Harbor Laboratory and the Harvard School of Public Health, proved invaluable in providing a background on the etiology of cancer.

Finally, I would like to thank my husband Stephen T. Whelan who took the time to read and appraise each version, and to the New York Academy of Medicine and New York Public Libraries for their courteous and efficient assistance in locating the vast quantity of research material which was vital to the preparation of this book.

Introduction

Perhaps a bumper sticker I saw recently said it all: "Life Causes Cancer." That slogan may well reflect the resignation to which many Americans have succumbed in the past few decades. Almost daily we read or hear about news reports of yet another "carcinogen" (cancer-causing agent) in the environment, or worse, on our dinner plate. This apparently all began with frightening tales about cranberries: they were conspicuously absent from America's Thanksgiving tables in 1959 because a government official announced that an herbicide used in the cranberry bogs caused cancer in rodents.

Then followed similar, unsettling headlines about the artificial sweeteners saccharin and cyclamates, Red Dye #2, nitrite used in curing bacon, hair dyes, the herbicide 2,4,5-T, dioxins, and the pesticide ethylene dibromide (EDB). News stories of the 1970s, 1980s and 1990s told us that we could get cancer from breathing city air, or develop leukemia, genetic damage, and more from living near nuclear or toxic waste dumps, using cellular phones, and even sleeping next to our alarm clocks. Others raised questions about the carcinogenic potential of specific, everyday foods and beverages like coffee, barbecued steaks, and apple juice. Still others pointed to the overall American diet as a leading cause of cancer death.

The explosion of news stories in the past twenty years about "carcinogens" in our food supply and general environment seems to have generated two different public reactions: first, that of resignation as summarized in the bumper sticker: second, one of anger—and demands for government action to "do something" to reduce our exposure to carcinogenic risks. We have seen our regulatory agencies—Environmental Protection Agency, Food and Drug Administration, Consumer Product Safety Commission, Occupational Safety and Health Administration—take aggressive action in an attempt to purge the land of man-made chemicals shown in the laboratory to cause cancer in animals. Self-appointed consumer groups such as the Ralph Nader-inspired Health Research Group, the Center for Science in the Public Interest, and the Natural Resources Defense Council seem committed to further pressuring the government to detect and purge the environment of synthetic animal carcinogens, all in an alleged effort to win the war against cancer.

Unfortunately, in the flurry of activity to ban pesticides, food additives and other synthetic compounds, one very important element has been missing: perspective. Obviously, if we are going to wage a successful war against cancer, we must begin by identifying the correct enemies. Certainly it would be futile for our society to invest dollars and personal energies in combatting hypothetical cancer risks while the known ones secure an even firmer grip upon us.

In *The Complete Guide to Preventing Cancer,* I will present, in layman's language, a full overview of what we know about the causes of human cancer, placing special emphasis on those causes over which we have some degree of control.

The information presented in this book is neither speculative nor based on my personal opinion. The contents that follow are reflective of the conclusions of mainstream cancer epidemiologists, and are almost exclusively based on the results of studies of human beings, as opposed to laboratory animals. In addition to doing a full literature review on the causes of human malignancies, I relied heavily on some of the state-of-the-art publications in this field, including the classic text by Sir Richard Doll and Richard Peto, *The Causes of Cancer,* originally published in the June 1981 edition of the *Journal of the National Cancer Institute; Cancer Epidemiology and Prevention,* edited by David Shottenfeld, M.D. (from the University of Michigan School of Public Health) and Joseph F. Fraumeni, M.D. (of the National Cancer Institute); *Cancer Rates and Risks,* a 1985 publication of the U.S. Department of Health and Human Services; and *Epidemiology and Health Risk Assessment,* a 1988 text edited by Leon Gordes.

This book is intended as a personal guide for you and your family. But it should do even more than that. When you finish reading the pages that follow you will have developed a new sophistication and skepticism about the phrase "cancer-causing agent." I hope this sophisticated skepticism will give you the perspective to react intelligently when the next chemical phobia seizes the nation, as it did in 1989 when millions of Americans threw away their apples, apple juice, and apple sauce after hearing about the alleged dangers of the agricultural chemical Alar.

Further, I hope you will come away with a full sense of the most significant preventive medicine reality of our time: *the more we learn about the causes of chronic diseases like cancer, the more we realize that much of our fate lies within our own hands.* While earlier generations could call upon government for regulations that would keep them healthy (chlorinating water, immunizing children), the state of knowledge about cancer as we approach the twenty-first century dictates that our regulatory agencies can do little or nothing to protect us. The key to cancer prevention lies within ourselves—and our lifestyles.

Dr. Elizabeth M. Whelan
New York City
April 1994

Part One

The Basics

1

Establishing the Causes
of Human Cancer

The word "cancer" generally describes a large group of diseases—perhaps as many as two hundred distinct entities—characterized by uncontrolled growth and the spread of abnormal cells. One or more of the body's cells apparently undergoes specific changes and can no longer function normally. A cell is generally thought to be cancerous when it grows and divides much more rapidly than do normal cells. Uncontrollable cancer growth can result in death.

A tumor is an abnormal mass of tissue that grows more rapidly than do normal tissues. *Benign* tumors generally grow slowly, do not spread, do not invade normal surrounding tissues, and rarely recur once removed. Even though they are not a form of cancer, benign tumors can damage surrounding tissues or organs by pressure if growth is extensive. *Malignant* tumors are made up of cancer cells that can multiply rapidly and threaten all body functions. They are capable of metastasizing, or spreading, to other tissues anywhere in the body. Cancer originating in the breast, for example, can metastasize to the brain. Through the process of metastasis, the entire body can become riddled with cancer.

Cancers probably long afflicted animals well before the human race appeared on earth. Evidence of cancer exists among mummies of the pre-Columbian Peruvian Incas, who lived some 2,400 years ago as determined by radioactive carbon dating. Hippocrates, the Greek philosopher and father of modern medicine, first gave cancer its name, based on the Greek word *karkinos,* meaning crab or ulcer. The capacity of cancer cells to invade and metastasize probably reminded Hippocrates of creeping, clutching crab claws, hence the origin of the word cancer.

How Does Cancer Originate?

Until this century, it was widely believed that cancer developed more or less spontaneously—that it was just a fact of life, or bad luck—and that there was very little that we could do to avoid the disease.

In fact there still remains some evidence that the onset of certain cancers is outside our control. Some cancer may be built into us as a part of our normal metabolism and may be related to the same process that causes aging. Numerous studies, both animal and human, confirm that the incidence of cancer dramatically increases with age (see chapter 2). However, only a small number of rare tumors have been proved to be directly related to genetic factors. Individuals with Down's syndrome have eleven times the normal risk of acute leukemia. A slightly increased risk of stomach cancer has been observed among individuals with blood group A.

In other rare instances, families have been identified with clusters of unusual kinds of cancers that seem to be genetically related. A white-skinned person is more likely to develop skin cancer with excessive sunlight exposure, as compared to a dark-skinned person.

On the other hand, epidemiological studies—that is, studies of human populations—have confirmed the critical importance of external causes of cancer in human beings. In other words, "nurture" as opposed to "nature" seems more important in cancer causation. Further, it now appears that there is no "one cause" of a given cancer, but a variety of circumstances, genetic as well as extrinsic (meaning external influences) that trigger the expression of cancer. In other words, there is a growing recognition that most cancers result from the combined effects of several circumstances and varying individual susceptibility.

"Environmentally Determined" Cancers

Epidemiology has long contributed to our knowledge about the causes of cancer. This approach dates back to 1700 when Bernardini Ramazzini (1713), the so-called "father of occupational hygiene," noted that breast-cancer rates were particularly elevated among nuns. He concluded that this increase was related to the fact that nuns do not marry. Only later was this association explained by childlessness (see chapter 7). In 1775 surgeon Percivall Pott noted that young chimney sweeps had an extraordinarily high frequency of scrotal cancer, which he associated with their daily occupational exposure to soot. Only centuries later did researchers determine that soot contains many carcinogenic hydrocarbons. Dr. John Hill, in 1761, noted an unusually high frequency of nasal cancer among snuff users, well before tobacco carcinogens were identified.

In recent times astute observers have noted an excessive number of patients with the same tumor and traced this "cluster" to a particular environmental exposure. The evidence that much of human cancer is avoidable can be derived from three specific sources:

1. *Differences in the incidence of cancer among human groups.* As will be elaborated upon in chapter 2, cancer frequency and type varies significantly from country to country. The range of variation is never less than sixfold and commonly much more. Liver cancer, for example, is common in parts of sub-Saharan Africa, but is rare in the United States. Breast cancer is common in the United States but rare in Japan, while stomach cancer is common there and uncommon here. Given that we are all human, this is clear evidence that cancer is not purely a human heredity disease, but is somewhat related to our environment, as defined by a broad spectrum of factors.

2. *Migrant studies.* The "environmental influence" hypothesis derived from international analysis of cancer frequency is reinforced by observations from migrant studies. Evidence of a change in the frequency of various cancers in groups that leave their homeland for residence in a new country provides further evidence of the importance of lifestyle or other environmental factors in the development of disease. The differences in rates between homeland and new country among identical ethnic groups leaves no doubt that new influencing factors—environmental factors—were

introduced with migration. Descendants of Japanese im-
migrants to the United States develop the cancer incidence
patterns typical of other Americans within one generation.
Persons of Scandinavian and Celtic descent have low rates
of skin cancer when living in Northern Europe, but persons
with the same ethnic background who live in tropical areas
have high skin-cancer rates, due to greater exposure to
sunlight.

Other groups for which data are available include Indians
who went to Fiji and South Africa (and thus no longer were
at high risk of developing oral cancers), and Britons who
went to Fiji (and acquired a high risk of skin cancer).

3. *Changes in cancer incidence over time.* Changes in the
frequency of particular types of cancer with the passage
of time provide conclusive evidence that the introduction
or removal of causal factors plays a causative or protective
role. A classic example is the observation that lung cancer
was a very rare disease in the United States in 1900. It
is now the leading cause of cancer death in American men
and has recently surpassed breast cancer as the leading cause
of cancer death in American women. In the United States,
stomach cancer was a common cause of cancer death early
in this century but it is now rare. Genetics cannot account
for such drastic changes in just a few generations, but
changing exposure to extrinsic cancer-causing agents or
patterns can.

How Much of Cancer Is Caused by the Environment?

It is currently estimated that between 75 and 80 percent of human cancer in the United States is attributable to extrinsic factors—or is traced to a person's environment—and hence is potentially preventable. Unfortunately, however, the definition of the term "environmental cancer" has been greatly distorted in recent years, leading many to believe that "environmental means man-made or industrial factors." This is not the case. The 75 to 80 percent figure, and its variations, has its origins in the work of Dr. John Higginson, founding director of the World Health Organization's International Agency for Research on Cancer. During the 1950s, Dr. Higginson compared the incidence of certain types of tumors among blacks in Africa and America and concluded that about two-thirds of all cancers had an environmental cause and were, therefore, at least theoretically preventable.

What desperately needs clarification is the word "environment": when used in identifying the causes of cancer, it means everything except heredity. Personal habits are therefore considered an "environmental factor," foremost among these being cigarette smoking. Other "environmental" causes of cancer include sunlight (responsible for almost all cases of superficial skin cancer); exposure to drugs like diethylstilbestrol (which caused a rare type of vaginal cancer in a small number of the daughters of mothers who used it during pregnancy); exposure to certain occupational factors (asbestos, vinyl chloride, among others); high-dose exposure to radiation; sexual and reproductive patterns (cervical cancer is more frequent among women who have multiple sexual partners; women who have their first child after age thirty, or have no children at all, are at somewhat higher risk of breast cancer than other women); and the broad components of our diet (we are still uncertain as to the exact relationship between specific dietary components and cancer risks).

Indeed, epidemiologists Doll and Peto in their classic, state-of-the-art review *Causes of Cancer* largely *dismiss* the notion that "environmental cancer" is related to pollution, toxic wastes, and "chemicals," emphasizing that while 25 to 40 percent of cancers are due to tobacco use, the best estimate of the contribution to cancer mortality by all types of pollution is 2 percent.

The new emphasis on environmentally caused cancers is a significant advance in our understanding of the etiology of the many diseases falling under the heading "cancer." But there have been some problems, particularly among lay people, in understanding the concepts of causation. Not only, as mentioned, has there been an unfortunate emphasis on "chemicals" as being synonymous with "environment," but the "80 percent of cancers are caused by the environment" statement has left many people with the unfounded belief that we should know the causes of all cancer that occur.

"What gave me my cancer?" is the typical question patients are now asking their doctors. Whereas in the past people tended to view malignant disease as a result of aging, heredity or bad luck, they now perceive cancer as a matter brought about exclusively by definable and controllable extrinsic forces. However, that is overstating our knowledge. It is within this context that some cancer patients and their families are striking out to blame their environment, the fact that they live near a chemical plant, or some specific type of food as the cause of their illness.

The reality is, however, that while we can feel justified

in claiming that the majority of cancers are environmentally related, we have only limited knowledge about what specific environmental factors are within our ability to manipulate. For example, while we might estimate that 35 percent of cancers in the United States are somehow related to diet, we simply do not know at this time what specific dietary factor is causal. Thus, when someone in this country develops colon cancer, he or she might demand to know what dietary component caused it. While research points us in specific directions, we haven't yet honed in on exacting relationships.

Cancer and Aging

Advancing age is the single most important risk factor for the development of cancer. Noted biochemist and cancer researcher Bruce N. Ames, Ph.D., has pointed out that the cumulative cancer risk increases with age, both in short-lived species such as rats and mice and in longer-lived species such as humans. About 30 percent of rats, mice, and humans have cancer by the end of their life span. Although scientists have not yet identified the exact mechanism responsible, something called immunosenescence may at least partially account for this increased cancer risk. Basically, immunosenescence means the body's immune system is less vigilant and the minor cellular changes that preface cancerous changes are not corrected. They thus progress to full-blown cancer.

How Do We Determine What Causes Cancer?

The rules by which disease causation can be proved developed gradually, beginning in the mid-nineteenth century.

The 1849 London cholera epidemic afforded an excellent opportunity to observe disease "cause and effect" in action. At that time the Germ Theory of disease causation had not yet been thought of, nor had bacteria been discovered, making accurate evaluation of the situation unlikely (if not impossible). Nevertheless, a doctor by the name of John Snow eventually put the pieces together correctly.

Snow noticed that victims came down with cholera in a seemingly haphazard fashion—some sections of London had clearly high cholera rates, others very low, and some intermediate. After ruminating upon this awhile, he looked into the community water supplies, since by that point in history cholera had been empirically associated with "bad water" (people saw a connection between dirty water and cholera, but didn't know why the association existed). Snow found that people living in some areas of London were supplied with water by the Southwark and Vauxhall Company, while other areas were supplied with water by the Lambeth Company. Through careful detective work, Snow discovered that certain other areas of London were supplied with water piped in from both water companies. What was more surprising was that each company ran pipes to houses in the same neighborhoods, and that there was no setting of boundaries between the companies' service areas. Because of this, people living on the same street, and perhaps even next door to one another, were supplied by different water companies.

As it turned out, the Southwark and Vauxhall Company

obtained its water from the Thames downstream, where it was contaminated with the offal of all mid-nineteenth-century London. The result: those people supplied with water from this company had high cholera rates. Geographically, cases appeared most often in areas supplied by both companies. As a result of Snow's careful investigation of the London water system, the "haphazard" distribution of cases was explained.

In true heroic fashion, Snow symbolically "stopped" the epidemic by taking away the handle of the Broad Street pump, which offered public access to the contaminated water. In truth, the epidemic was already on the wane, but Snow's dramatic and perceptive connections between cholera, geographic area, and the key "risk factor"—exposure to water from the guilty company—remains a classic introduction to proof of causation.

By the end of the nineteenth century, microorganisms had been discovered and most, if not all, doctors accepted the idea that some diseases—what would be termed infectious diseases—were caused by microorganisms. Bacteriologist Robert Koch developed a list of criteria to prove causation in human disease. The list included such concepts as:

1. Exposure to the "causative" agent must precede disease.

2. To prove an organism caused disease, first it had to be isolated from someone with the illness, reintroduced into another subject, and the disease had to reappear in the new subject.

3. The organism in question should not have been found in those without the disease.

Koch's postulates worked very well for infectious diseases, and indeed they still do (although they are difficult to apply to viruses). But when it comes to applying the postulates to human chronic diseases that are not caused by microorganisms—such as heart attacks, arthritis, and cancer—Koch's postulates fall short. Obviously, for these diseases, there has to be some other way to establish their causes.

Sir Austin Bradford Hill in 1964 updated Koch's guidelines, noting once again that for infectious agents Koch's postulates were very relevant. But for noninfectious agents, he suggested this set of guidelines for establishing causation:

1. *Strength of association:* Strong associations are likely to be causal, but the fact that an association is weak does not rule out a causative relationship. By strength of association, Hill refers to the magnitude of the ratio of incidences. His argument is essentially that strong associations are likely to be causal, because if they were due to confounding or some other bias, the biasing association would have to be even stronger and would therefore presumably be more evident. Weak associations are more likely to be explained by biases, but the fact that an association is weak does not rule out a causal connection.

2. *Consistency:* Consistency refers to replication in different populations under different circumstances, but a factor may be causal without being consistent. That is, lack of consistency does not rule out a causal association, because some effects are produced by their causes only under unusual circumstances.

3. *Specificity:* This criterion refers to the requirement that a cause should lead to a single effect. However, an event in reality may have many different effects. For example, smoking causes many diseases other than lung cancer.

4. *Temporality:* The cause must *always* precede the effect in time.

5. *Biologic gradient:* This criterion refers to the presence of a dose-response curve. Some causal associations, however, show no apparent trend of effect with dose; an example is the association between diethylstilbestrol and adenocarcinoma of the vagina. A possible explanation is that the doses of diethylstilbestrol administered were all sufficiently great to produce the maximum effect, with actual development of disease depending on other component causes.

6. *Plausibility and Coherence:* The supposed causal relationship has to be consistent with known existing biological facts—and have some possible biological hypothesis underlying it. For example, constant irritation of the lungs with carcinogen-containing smoke clearly presents a biologically plausible explanation of lung cancer.

The biological hypotheses that attempt to explain apparent increased risk are not always as straightforward as the lung-cancer smoking link. Recent evidence indicates that smokers are at increased risk of cervical cancer. No immediate biological connection comes to mind here, but laboratory data do suggest that cigarette smoke and its components permeate the body, including the reproductive tract.

What Types of Data and Study Methodologies Are Used to Determine the Causes of Cancer?

There are three different procedures available to the scientific community to evaluate the role of extrinsic factors in the causation of cancer: *epidemiology,* or the study of human populations; *animal testing;* and *short term assays.* These three types of investigations provide evidence that a substance is or is not associated with cancer. None actually *proves* that a particular substance is responsible for cancer. Causation is a very difficult thing to prove for potential carcinogens, since long periods of time may pass between exposure and development of the disease. So instead of trying to prove something *causes* cancer, in the traditional use of the word "cause," scientists attempt to demonstrate that exposure to substances or lifestyle factors *increase the likelihood of getting cancer.* If an agent does increase the risk, it strengthens the case for causation.

Epidemiology

Epidemiological studies investigate the effects that suspected carcinogens or lifestyles have had or will have on human cancer. The first indication that an epidemiological study is appropriate usually comes from what might be called a "red flag"—the observation that certain clusters of people seem to have unusually high rates of a particular kind of cancer. In a preliminary investigation, scientists might find a similar group of people without the cancer in question, and compare the two groups for exposure to unusual factors that might have caused the disease. This type of study is called a case-control, or retrospective study, because it starts out with people who have already developed cancer and "goes back in history" to find out what may have caused it. In this manner, epidemiologists can ascertain "risk factors" for the cancer in question. Better evidence that these risk factors actually cause cancer (rather than being merely associated with it) comes from prospective epidemiological studies. In a prospective, or longitudinal study, the researchers start out with a group of people who do not have cancer, but can be separated into exposure groups, that is, one group exposed to the suspected agent, one group not. The observers watch the groups over a period of time to see if the exposure groups develop more cancer—for example, if smokers develop more cancers than nonsmokers. The prospective study offers stronger evidence of cause-effect because it assures that exposure preceded the disease.

Epidemiology has the great virtue of directly identifying *human* risk factors, and hence it does not suffer from the same kinds of uncertainties of interpretation that are associated with animal tests. Many chemicals and industrial processes have been found by this means to cause human cancer. The International Agency for Research on Cancer (IARC) recently reported eighteen such causes, in addition to cigarette smoking, alcohol, and radiation, which had already been identified as cancer-causing agents. The same report also listed an additional eighteen "probable" causes of human cancer. Another recent survey identified some forty risk factors for various human cancers, including lifestyle factors such as "late age at first pregnancy," "sexual promiscuity," "obesity," and certain infectious diseases, including AIDS, hepatitis B, and various parasites.

Epidemiology suffers from several inherent defects, however. It is difficult to establish small effects with statistical confidence by epidemiological means. "Small," in this case, means proportionately small; an effect that could not be confirmed by an epidemiologic study of a limited group of people might still be responsible for a significant number of cases of disease each year in a larger population.

One problem in epidemiologic studies is the difficulty of assembling reliable information on large numbers of people by means of interviews or examination of medical records. It is also not easy to find groups of people to compare who differ *only* in the single factor under study. If they differ in other ways, these other differences, called "confounding variables," might generate a spurious relationship or conceal a true one. This is often a problem even when the effect under investigation is large, but when it is at most small, such as the hypothetical effect of saccharin on bladder cancer or of hair dyes on breast cancer, the problem can be insurmountable.

It is particularly difficult to find comparison groups of people who have never been exposed to the factor under study (zero-dose control groups). For example, if we wanted to test the hypothesis that caffeine caused cancer, it would be almost impossible to find a sizable group of people with no exposure to caffeine at all, since caffeine is a constituent of coffee, tea, cola beverages, and some other drinks; cocoa and chocolate products; and many over-the-counter drugs. We would have to look at special groups of people such as Seventh Day Adventists, who make a deliberate effort to abstain from major sources of caffeine (such as coffee). However, groups of this type differ from the general population in many other ways, so we would then be faced with many possible confounding variables.

Epidemiological studies led to the very important discovery that cancer can first appear decades *after* initial exposure to a carcinogenic substance. Such cancers are said to have a long latency period. For instance, cigarette smokers don't usually develop lung cancer sooner than twenty years after they start smoking. Similarly, lung cancers in asbestos workers typically develop several decades after the first exposure to asbestos. Some of the daughters of women who were given the drug diethylstilbestrol (DES) during pregnancy have developed vaginal cancer. These cancers only became manifest after the daughters passed puberty, many years following the actual exposure to the drug.

Such long latency periods are another factor that makes epidemiological investigations of cancer causation difficult, because the search for causes of current cancer cases must focus on events that took place several decades in the past. Memories of these events have faded and records have often been lost.

Moreover, these long latencies mean that one must wait for decades to establish that a current or recent exposure will or will not result in cancer in the future. Thus, human studies cannot assess the effects of the many new chemicals constantly generated by a modern industrial economy— about a thousand each year in the United States alone— until sufficient time has elapsed. Since the toxic effects, including cancer, of such new chemicals must be identified before significant human exposure to them can be allowed, alternative testing methods must be used.

About Animal Testing

Many of our cancer alarms, including the Alar-apple scam, cyclamates, and red dye #2, come from the same source: tests in laboratory animals which lead to pronouncements that the substance tested could cause cancer in humans. The results of these tests affect all of us. Our health and standard of living depend on decisions based on these tests. The availability of products that we use everyday depends on them. Billions of dollars in pollution controls, insurance premiums, product changes and modifications, damage payments, and legal fees depend upon the results of animal tests and their interpretation.

Is this heavy reliance on animal cancer testing justified? Are the results of such tests truly applicable to human health? There are good reasons to ask these questions. Recent scientific controversy has emphasized the limitations of animal cancer testing and its relevance to human cancer hazard.

Most Americans first became aware of this issue when the U.S. Food and Drug Administration (FDA) declared the artificial sweetener saccharin to be a carcinogen in 1977. This determination rested on tests that showed the artificial sweetener could cause tumors in rats under conditions of massive, prolonged exposure. Cancer frequently increased only when saccharin was administered in amounts equivalent to the consumption by a human of about 1,000 cans of diet soda a day, beginning with the weaning of the parent generation of rats, and continuing throughout the conception, gestation, nursing, and adult lifetime of the animals that ultimately developed tumors. Even under these extreme conditions, only male rats in the second generation developed tumors and only one organ was affected (the bladder) with no metastasis (spreading to other sites) or otherwise lethal tumors observed. Many people who are aware of these facts question whether the result really demonstrates that human consumption of ordinary amounts of saccharin poses a significant cancer hazard, particularly since epidemiological studies of long-term high frequency users of saccharin (e.g., diabetics) show no increase in bladder cancer.

On the other hand, U.S. health and safety regulatory agencies consistently assure the public that, despite the uncertainties, the results of such animal tests are valid and provide a sound basis for decisions about human hazard. The zeal to publicize results from animal studies on carcinogenicity reached its zenith in the mid-1970s when the National Cancer Institute (NCI) issued their "Memorandum of Alert" whenever a bioassay of a chemical in rats or mice showed a cancer response. The results often appeared in the news media long before publication in a scientific journal. Many scientists viewed these news releases with skepticism as "the carcinogen of the week." Currently, the NCI/ National Toxicology Program (NTP) testing program, in collaboration with regulatory agencies, generally presents a more careful evaluation before there is a public alert.

In light of these drawbacks, you may be wondering why researchers continue to use animal tests. First, there are many limitations to population-based, or epidemiological, studies, as discussed earlier. Second, animal tests, when used and interpreted properly, can assist in predicting human cancer risk.

The History of Animal Testing

The first demonstration that cancer could be induced in animals by treating them with chemicals was in 1915. Early studies tested presumed potent carcinogenic chemicals to discover mechanism of action, metabolic fates, and other attributes. Such studies were expanded in the early 1960s to become routine bioassays on a whole series of selected chemicals.

During the 1970s preliminary tests indicated that mutagenicity (ability to cause genetic damage) could be correlated with carcinogenicity and that the presence of certain chemical structures suggested potential carcinogenicity (e.g., aromatic amines and polycyclic compounds). The extent of human exposure, whether occupational or environmental, also affected the selection of chemicals for testing.

The early selection process for chemical carcinogenicity studies favored chemicals that are thought to be significant carcinogens, i.e., the ratio of chemicals being positive to those producing no response was purposely chosen to be high. Indeed, this has continued to be the practice. The National Cancer Institute adopted this initial selection design and the National Toxicology Program (NTP), which later took over the bioassay program, now uses essentially the same design.

How Are Standard Animal Cancer Tests Performed?

A standard test is performed on both sexes of two species of animals, chiefly rats and mice. These animals are chosen because they are less expensive to maintain than other mammals. The animals are exposed to the test substance for most or all of their lives (about two years) to maximize the chances of detecting cancers, most of which have long latency periods.

The selected route of exposure to the substance generally matches as closely as possible the route of human exposure. Chemicals are injected by intra-muscular, intraperitoneal, intravenous, and subcutaneous routes. Test materials in solution may be painted on the skin or exposure may be through inhalation, in drinking water, or in the diet. Unpalatable substances are given by stomach tube.

There are various experimental conditions for dosing, patterns of dosing, and time frames of observations. The procedures (protocols) for pathological examinations for tumors, both benign and malignant, also have varied. Some studies examine more organs than others and the thoroughness of tissue examination can differ.

The standard bioassay now uses three dose groups in rats and mice. The control group does not receive the chemical but is otherwise identical to the other three dose groups. The "high," "mid," or "low" dose groups receive the chemicals at different dose levels. Fifty animals make up each sex/species/dose group for a total of 800 animals in four sex-species experiments. Before the cancer study is performed, preliminary range-finding experiments determine the proper dose levels. Upon study completion, pathologists examine thousands of microscopic slides of some of the tissues and organs from each animal to detect tumors that might be invisible to the naked eye. The whole procedure for testing and evaluation of one chemical takes three or more years to complete at a cost of about $1500 per animal or $1,000,000 for a typical test on a single material.

With only 800 animals, a relatively weak carcinogen is

likely to escape identification as cancer causing. A substance would have to induce cancer in about 7 to 10 percent of the exposed animals in order for there to be a good chance of detecting its carcinogenic action with statistical confidence in a test of this size. If spontaneous tumors appear in the control animals (as commonly occurs) as well as the test group, then the test would be even less sensitive. In theory, one could design a test involving a much larger number of animals that could detect weak carcinogens, but increasing the number of animals greatly increases the cost. Experiments with very large numbers of animals are logistically difficult to perform because it is difficult to keep track of large numbers of animals at each stage in the experiment. For the purpose of testing sizable numbers of chemicals simply to see whether they might be carcinogenic, the NCI/NTP size test is about as large as is practical.

How Large Are the Dosages Used in These Tests?

In order to compensate for the limited number of animals tested, large dosages are used to try to detect even a weak carcinogen. The rationale is that, in general, the incidence of tumors will increase as the dose of carcinogen becomes larger.

The Maximum Tolerated Dose (MTD) is the largest estimated dose that the animals can tolerate without a 10 percent weight loss compared to controls. In some instances, injury can also occur. It is standard practice in animal cancer bioassays to use the MTD as the highest test dose in a typical animal cancer test. The "low" dose is usually one-half or one-fourth of the MTD—still a very high dose compared to most human exposure. The belief that using the MTD will maximize the power of animal tests to detect weak carcinogens is the principal reason why regulatory agencies use animal cancer test results as "valid" indicators of presumed human carcinogenicity.

These MTDs are usually many orders of magnitude—thousands or millions of times—above the dose humans encounter. Table 1 compares the doses of test chemicals given to rodents with the equivalent intake which a human would have to ingest to equal the rodent dose. Clearly, the enormous doses in many animal studies are not equivalent to a typical human exposure. Yet, these animal studies still form the basis for regulatory action.

Two of the chemicals listed—the nonnutritive sweeteners saccharin and cyclamates—were regulated based on the results of high-dose animal studies. FDA banned cyclamates in 1970 under the Delaney Amendment to the Food, Drug and Cosmetic Act. Safrole and its equivalent sassafras were banned as flavoring agents because of their classification as an animal carcinogen. Diethylstilbestrol (DES) was originally used in the prevention of spontaneous abortion, but this use no longer is approved by the FDA, because in certain animal species long term DES administration increases the frequency of certain cancers and because in women DES and other natural and synthetic estrogens have been linked to endometrial cancer. (DES now is used cautiously to treat metastatic breast cancer in women and in metastatic prostate cancer in men.) DES was given to cattle as a growth stimulant but FDA halted this use many years ago.

Table 1.1
Comparative Animal/Human Doses
for Selected Chemicals

Chemical	Experimental Daily Dose (rodents unless noted)	Equivalent Human Intake
Cyclamates	5% in diet (2.18 gms/day)	138–522 12 oz. bottles of soda (daily) or about 80–240 times typical human intake.
Saccharin	0.5, 5.0, or 7.5% in diet[a]	40–400 times daily human intake or up to 500 times typical consumption of sweeteners[b]
DES	One clinical treatment[c]	5 million pounds of beef liver from treated cattle for 50 years
Safrole	5,000 ppm in diet (0.5%)	613 12 oz. bottles of root beer daily
Alar[d]	5,000–10,000 ppm in diet (0.5 to 1.0%)	28,000 pounds of apples daily for 10 years

a. Only a few bladder tumors found for high-dose animals. European studies at 0.5% intake produced no tumors.

b. Average sugar consumption is about 150 grams per day. A saccharin dose of 3.75 mg. per day per kg. body weight is equivalent to the sweetness of 135 kg. of sucrose or sugar per day.

c. The experimental dose refers to the clinical DES dose to women not an animal dose.

d. Alar (daminozide) is a plant growth regulator that improves apple texture, appearance, crispness, and storage characteristics.

How Much Do Animal Cancer Tests Cost?
Are They a Cost-Effective Means to
Protect Human Health?

A lifetime study on a chemical in the rodent bioassay costs about $1,000,000. However, social costs calculated for the misclassification of chemical substances should be included in any evaluation. False classification of a chemical as a carcinogen means it may never be marketed in developed countries. If this chemical is of high value to society, then its replacement or abandonment eliminates the benefit. In addition, engineering controls for minimizing the exposure to a chemical which, in reality, is a noncarcinogen increases the manufacturing cost for the substance and consequently its cost to consumers is increased.

Including the social costs in the cost for the bioassay gives estimates in the range of millions of dollars. Such overall estimates include the costs for misclassification and the designation of false positives and false negatives, costs far higher for screening bioassays than for screening a chemical on the basis of short term tests. For this reason some investigators conclude that the rodent bioassay is not cost-effective for most chemicals.

In the last decade scientists began to raise objections to the broad utilization of such screening tests. The bioassay screening declares a chemical to be an animal carcinogen based on a positive response in one or more species. This may not be sufficient to designate a chemical as a carcinogenic hazard to human beings.

Critics argued that more research was needed on metabolism associated with different dosing regimens. In addition, bioassays could be modified to reveal more useful information on the metabolic fate (pharmacokinetics) of the chemical as administered to rodents over a graduated range of doses, a procedure that would be more relevant to exposure levels and modes in the human population. For example, it would make more sense to use skin painting for hair dyes than to use oral feeding of such chemicals to test animals. Extending the bioassay protocol toward pharmacokinetic evaluation and more applicable administration routes could improve the utility of animal studies in the health assessment process.

Commonly used chemicals number about 60,000 and only a few are potent, recognized carcinogens. Yet today's regulatory processes require that chemicals or drugs be subjected to extensive testing before they are marketed or manufactured. Based on animal carcinogenicity tests, one would expect a high ratio of test chemicals to turn up positive, because about 65 percent of the 800 chemicals tested have shown some carcinogenic activity in animals.

Since animal carcinogenicity tests appear to be the "gold standard" to approve or reject chemicals, the lack of consistency between recognized human carcinogens and the high percentage of tested chemicals with carcinogenic activity in animals needs to be recognized. For many chemicals there is no consistency between the effects observed in mice compared to that seen in rats. When a test chemical in the bioassay shows a broad carcinogenic response in multiple species over a spectrum of doses, then there is a good concordance in responses. However, when there is a lack of concordance, as for example in the response of rats as compared to mice, then the test result is less clear. Frequently, one faces false positives and false negatives in the test results.

Have Animal Cancer Tests Ever Successfully Predicted Carcinogenicity in Humans?

Yes, there have been seven cases in which chemicals first found to be animal carcinogens in one or more species were later discovered to be human carcinogens. The substances are aflatoxin, 4-amino-biphenyl, DES, bis(chloromethyl)-ether, melphalan, mustard gas, and vinyl chloride. Currently, several hundred chemicals are classified as carcinogens on the basis of animal tests. However, one cannot pick the seven vindicated as human carcinogens to argue that animal tests in general are excellent predictors of human cancer risk.

There are hundreds of chemicals classified as "carcinogens" in at least one animal test for which it has not been possible to establish that the substance also causes human cancer. DDT, saccharin, and cyclamates are examples and there are many more. Often epidemiological studies show that the exposed populations have much less cancer than would be expected if the animal studies were correct.

There is insufficient evidence to argue persuasively that animal cancer tests, as currently conducted and evaluated, can confidently predict whether a given substance will cause human cancer.

This situation is unfortunate because regulatory officials suggest that they are left with little choice but to resolve all uncertainties in interpreting animal cancer tests by assuming the worst in each instance. The extreme assumptions arising from this orientation include: (1) use of the MTD so as not to miss "weak" carcinogens; (2) the assumption that risk is linearly related to dose even when the studies show otherwise; (3) using the results from the most susceptible species, strain, and sex as the basis for inferring human risk even when negative results in other test animals abound; (4) ignoring the experience of decades of safe human use, or other negative evidence; (5) counting benign tumors as though they were as significant as malignant tumors; (6) many similar decisions made in an effort to be as "prudent" as possible; and (7) ignoring the level of human exposure, which generally is a very small percentage of animal exposure in the laboratory.

The compounded impact of these choices is to bias the analysis of animal tests only in the direction of concluding that the substance in question is an animal carcinogen. Since there is no obvious way of discovering when a prediction of human cancer risk based on a positive judgment in an animal test is incorrect, we cannot measure the effect that this deliberate bias has on the frequency of false positive judgments. With a high rate of false positives, the identification of truly dangerous substances may be swamped by false positives, and the ability of regulatory agencies to make discriminating policy decisions—i.e., identifying and controlling risks that matter—is severely hindered.

Are There Other Procedures Instead of the Rodent Bioassay for Carcinogenicity?

Yes, biomedical scientists are devoting extensive research efforts to developing short-term tests to replace laboratory animals. These short-term studies include bacterial systems and tissue cultures. In addition, there are efforts to use lower forms of life such as chick embryos and small fish or to use computer simulations and structure activity studies.

Short-term bioassays using bacterial systems, for example, are capable of showing that a specific chemical is a mutagen or is genotoxic. The best known short-term test is the Ames test using Salmonella typhimurium, a bacterium that is challenged with a candidate chemical in a laboratory growth medium. Often chemicals that are mutagens appear to be carcinogens, but not all chemicals identified as carcinogens are necessarily mutagens. It is the epigenetic carcinogens—those that alter the expression of genes without affecting the genes themselves—that may thwart the Ames test, because they do not interact with genetic material in the test.

Animal studies with nonhuman primates (monkeys or chimpanzees, etc.) are, in principle, quite valuable in sorting out discrepancies in bioassay results, since the nonhuman primate is likely to be a much more reliable predictor of human response to the substance under study. For example, early studies on saccharin using rodents produced some positive findings, but tests with monkeys over a span of twenty years found that saccharin did not generate tumors.

The use of small aquarium-type fish, such as the guppy, the Japanese medaka, the sheepshead minnow, and the rivulus, could possibly replace the use of the rodent for bioassay. These fish can be reared and maintained easily and economically in tanks in large numbers under carefully controlled conditions.

One advantage of fish over rodents is that the baseline is a low background prevalence of specific types of inducible tumors (essentially zero) for the control group of fish. This is in particular contrast with the mouse where there is a finite tumor incidence (spontaneous tumor incidence) in the control group of unchallenged animals. A low spontaneous tumor incidence suggests that any increase in observed incidence in the fish model exposed to a chemical practically reflects the number of tumors induced by the chemical without being confounded by background tumors.

With a large number of fish available in the tanks, it is possible to conduct extensive dose-response studies. Because the fish are sensitive to challenge with chemicals, the fish model also has the advantage of demonstrating a tumor response in several months rather than years for rodents. The maximum time for induced tumors in fish is no greater than one year after exposure. Studies with chlorinated compounds, representative of drinking-water contaminants, showed a dose-response curve with a threshold for a previously characterized carcinogen. Of course, fish are more distantly related to humans than small mammals like rats and mice; however, it is conceivable that the fish model could replace the rodent for routine bioassay studies.

2

A Cancer Epidemic?

A commonly held belief is that the United States is experiencing a cancer "epidemic." (An epidemic may be defined as a significant increase in the frequency of a disease.) However, with a few exceptions, most notably lung cancer, a careful inspection of the data currently available on cancer rates reveals that this is not the case. There has been little change in overall cancer mortality for at least the last forty years, although fluctuations have occurred for some individual types of cancers. In the case of cancer, what is excessive can be determined by a comparison of cancer rates over time, among different countries, and even among different groups within the same country. As will be seen, such comparisons do not reveal an overall cancer epidemic in the United States today.

Before looking at these comparisons we need to gain a working knowledge of how cancer statistics are typically calculated and the limitations of the sources from which they are obtained.

Ways of Looking at Cancer Data: Terminology

An important concept in cancer epidemiology is *incidence*—the number of new cases diagnosed in a given geographic area during a specific period of time. To compensate for variations in number of inhabitants in different areas, incidence is divided by the total population to yield the *incidence rate*. The measure thus formed is not influenced by population size and can be used for comparison.

Another important concept is cancer *mortality* or *death*. This is how many people in a given geographic place, during a specified period of time, die of cancer. Usually, one wants to compare cancer deaths, and therefore calculates *mortality* or *death rates* by dividing the number of deaths by the total population of the geographic location.

Theoretically, epidemiologists prefer incidence rates to death rates. Incidence rates are more closely associated with the occurrence of a disease and its causes. Incidence may also provide an important measure of the current success in preventing new cancers. By contrast, mortality data are the end result of the disease and are therefore further removed from its causes. Such data are also influenced by changes and advances in treatment. However, death rates for cancer are more readily available than incidence rates, because the cause of death appears on every death certificate. Thus, epidemiologists frequently use cancer death rates to indicate incidence rates. Death rates most closely resemble the incidence rates when the average survival time for a form of cancer is short. For example, lung cancer is one instance where incidence and death rates are similar.

Despite the theoretically valid argument just outlined, some evidence points to the unreliability of incidence rates for studying recent trends in cancer. With respect to some cancers, recent trends show either sharp increases or substantial fluctuations from year to year. The following sections deal with the "biases" (or systematic departures from true values) believed responsible for these statistical artifacts.

Occasionally, incidence rates and death rates are standardized or "adjusted" for an additional factor, namely age. The adjusted rate is composed of a weighted average of weights for specific age groups. The amount of weight given to each age group is determined by reference to a standard population. Since the risk of cancer increases with age and people in the United States are living longer today, failure to either adjust cancer rates by age can convey the impression of an overall increase in cancer when in fact there is none. Therefore, when one compares cancer rates over time, between places, or among racial and ethnic groups, where the age distribution varies, one generally adjusts the rates statistically to a standardized age distribution to make them comparable. Thus, changes in cancer frequency over and above those influenced by a changing age distribution become detectable.

Some researchers, however, believe that the study of age-specific trends in cancer mortality and incidence serves a unique purpose. If one wishes to assess the effect of recent changes in treatments and the effects of "carcinogenic" agents, an evaluation of the trends seen in the younger groups is particularly relevant.

Incidence rates and death rates are often reported per 100,000 persons. Also, it is common to report rates for a one-year period corresponding to a given calendar year.

The United States

Sources of Cancer Data

In the United States there is one primary source of data for incidence rates and one for death rates.

The National Cancer Institute (NCI) has conducted surveys of cancer incidence in the past (1937, 1947, 1969–71). It was not until 1973, however, that it began to constantly monitor cancer incidence through the Surveillance, Epidemiology and End Results (SEER) Program. This program involves collection of data from cancer registries in different geographic areas. The areas presently covered are the entire states of Connecticut, Hawaii, Iowa, New Mexico, and Utah. Also included are metropolitan Atlanta, Detroit, and the San Francisco-Oakland and Seattle-Puget Sound areas. The areas covered by SEER have changed slightly over the years.

Mortality data on cancer comes from the National Center for Health Statistics (NCHS) and are obtained from death certificates throughout the United States. Such data have been available since 1933.

Every year the American Cancer Society (ACS) uses data from the NCI and NCHS to compile estimates of both cancer incidence and mortality for the upcoming year. The annual ACS publication presenting this information is called *Cancer Facts and Figures.*

Accuracy

All three sources of cancer data have limitations, some of which are inherent in the data and can cause bias during examination of statistics for a specified period. In other circumstances, biases cause concern when we compare data from different time periods. Different kinds of degree of bias may characterize each period.

The major limitation of the recent NCI data (SEER) is that the geographic areas covered in the survey may not represent the United States as a whole, but were chosen because they represent epidemiologically diverse populations. Information included for incidence rates by site, age, race, and ethnicity allows epidemiologists to monitor changes in incidence over time and make comparisons among groups. In fact, mortality rates by cancer site, for the SEER areas and the United States as a whole, correspond closely, especially for whites. Thus, cancer incidence rates by site obtained from SEER may be representative for the white population.

In comparing incidence rates over time for NCI data, a number of important biases are relevant. First, there has been a change in the geographic areas covered. Although some overlap occurs among the first three NCI studies and the areas covered by SEER, there is also a significant difference in the areas covered by the earlier studies compared to those covered by SEER. A second bias stems from difference in the accuracy of area population estimates at different time periods. Another important problem likely to have varied over time lies in the care taken to include each cancer patient only once in the study and to include only new cases of cancer for the period under study. Accompanying this is the bias introduced by changes in the effort and motivation of physicians in registering cases of cancer incidence. Furthermore, over the years there have been technical changes in the definition of exactly what constitutes a cancer as well as changes in the methods and ability to diagnose many forms of the disease. Many experts believe that current cancer incidence rates are being inflated by a significant number of "over diagnoses"—growths that are biologically malignant but do not spread quickly and threaten the individual's health. In a previous report, the National Cancer Advisory Board identified this problem as inflating some cancer rates.

Data on death rates from the National Center for Health Statistics (NCHS) are subject to several kinds of problems. Since the source of these data (death certificates) has remained constant, biases in current data and those arising from comparisons with past data will be discussed together.

Rules governing the registration of deaths from one state to another may vary over time, thus introducing a source of bias and making comparisons more difficult. Classification systems used in the reporting of deaths have varied over time. Even when the exact type of cancer is detected while the patient is alive, the correct information may not appear on the death certificate. In addition, often only one underlying cause of death appears on a death certificate, and therefore some cancer deaths are incorrectly attributed to secondary causes or even missed entirely. Such errors are more likely to occur in elderly patients, and have been more of a problem in the past than now. In cases where the patient has widespread cancer, the primary site of the disease may not be known and/or properly recorded and thus the type of cancer is not specified on the death certificate. When cancer has spread, the death certificate may contain incorrect information as to its primary source. Sometimes a misdiagnosis of the cell type of cancer occurs. Many such errors can also affect incidence rates.

The annual *Cancer Facts and Figures* from the American Cancer Society (ACS) is a major source of cancer information disseminated to the public. It is thus fair to ask if the estimates of cancer death and incidence contained in this publication are accurate.

Because it takes time to compile nationwide information from death certificates, the ACS uses death rates three to five years old to project trends for the coming year. In general, their track record has been very good. One previous study found that when actual data become available and are compared to ACS estimates for specific sites, estimates were off by only two to four percent. The more common the type of cancer, the better the estimate tends to be. Estimates for sites with rapidly changing mortality (i.e., lung cancer in women) have been consistently low.

ACS estimates of incidence tend to be less accurate than death estimates, partly because actual rates from which estimates are made are limited to locations covered by SEER. Yet, estimates for incidence rates are made for the whole country. These estimates are also dependent upon the accuracy of population and mortality projections, which may contain errors. Incidence estimates for states covered by SEER, and for cancer sites, have been in error by as much as 22.3 percent, though, in fairness, they have also been within one percent of actual figures. However, it is not uncommon for these figures to be off by 15 to 20 percent.

One problem with all of the above sources of data is their comparability. For example, the ACS often report data in actual numbers rather than rates, while the SEER and NCHS figures are reported as rates. In addition, when rates are adjusted by age they are not necessarily standardized to the same base population. This creates additional error. Thus, comparisons of cancer statistics between publications or over time must be made with caution.

Time Trends in the United States

OVERALL INCIDENCE AND MORTALITY COMPARISONS

An important way of examining the issue of whether there is a cancer epidemic in the United States today is to look at patterns over time for cancers of specific sites. A comparison of the relative changes over time in both incidence and mortality rates can prove useful. Table 1 provides such a comparison between incidence and mortality for various cancer sites. As illustrated in the table, certain forms of cancer have had dramatic increases in incidence in recent years without a corresponding increase in mortality. Such changes may be due largely to increased screening for the disease.

A careful evaluation of Table 1 reveals that mortality caused by Hodgkin's disease and cancers of the cervix, uterus (endometrium), stomach, rectum, testis, bladder, thyroid, oral cavity, and pharynx has declined more than 15 percent since 1973.

Increases in mortality of greater than 15 percent have occurred since 1973 for lung cancer, melanoma, non-Hodgkin's lymphoma, and multiple myeloma. Lung cancer mortality rates support the evidence of an epidemic of lung cancer in the United States. Smoking has long been implicated as the cause of these elevated rates of lung cancer. Increases in cigarette smoking from 1900 until the 1960s transformed

Table 2.1
Cancer Sites Ranked by Percentage Change in Mortality and Incidence between 1973 and 1987 Based on Rates per 100,000 Age-adjusted to the 1970 U.S. Standard Population

Cancer Site or Type	Percentage Change, 1973–1975	
	Mortality	Incidence
Greater than 15% decrease in mortality and incidence		
Hodgkin's disease	−49.5	−15.9
Cervix	−39.6	−36.4
Stomach	−29.4	−36.4
Uterus (endometrium)	−19.8	−26.1
Greater than 15% decrease in mortality with increasing incidence		
Testis	−60.0	39.0
Rectum	−39.9	−3.3
Bladder	−22.7	12.3
Thyroid	−20.6	14.6
Oral cavity and pharynx	−16.2	−1.3
Greater than 15% increase in incidence with smaller change in mortality		
Kidney	12.9	27.0
Brain and other nervous system	9.4	23.0
Prostate	7.2	45.9
Breast	2.2	24.2
Fairly stable mortality and incidence		
Esophagus	11.3	12.3
Ovary	−6.4	−6.8
Larynx	−6.0	0.5
Leukemia	−5.6	−10.2
Liver	−4.7	14.5
Pancreas	−2.0	−5.6
Colon	−1.6	10.6
All sites	−5.4	14.6

Source: B. K. Henderson, et al., *Science* 254 (22 November 1993): 1131–37.

the once rare disease to the current leading cause of cancer death. The increase in melanoma parallels a larger increase in the incidence of the disease. This trend is mainly caused by overexposure to the sun in fair-skinned individuals. The increases in the incidence and mortality of non-Hodgkin's lymphoma and multiple myeloma may be due to improved diagnosis in the detection of the disease. As will be discussed later in this report, in younger age groups, much of the recent increased incidence of these diseases may be attributed to the increasing prevalence of human immunodeficiency virus infection (HIV), which is known to be associated with these forms of cancer.

Cancer of the breast and prostate have both increased in incidence, without a correspondingly large change in mortality. Early detection of these diseases, as well as increased utilization of screening procedures such as mammography, the digital rectal exam, and the prostate specific antigen (PSA) test can largely explain these trends. The 20 percent increase in the incidence of brain and other central nervous (CNS) tumors may be explained by the increased availability of x-ray computerized tomography in the diagnosis of previously undetected tumors. Some theorize that the increase in CNS tumor incidence may be the result of the exposure to dental x-rays. Specifically, the earlier forms of equipment resulted in much higher exposure than can be seen today. The increase in kidney cancer incidence and the lesser increase in mortality can be at least partially attributed to cigarette smoking.

Changes in mortality and incidence since 1973 have remained fairly stable for most of the remaining forms of cancer. However, the increases in esophagus and liver cancer can be largely explained by the combined effects of alcohol and tobacco.

Incidence: Specific Trends

The availability of data on incidence rates over time is limited. As mentioned earlier, before the SEER program, nationwide NCI cancer studies were used. Using two of these points in time (1947–50 and 1969–71) and the SEER results, the trends presented in Figures 1 and 2 emerge.

Of particular interest in Figures 1 and 2 are the changes in incidence rates seen in lung, breast, and prostate cancer. Although not illustrated in Figure 1 due to limited data points, male lung cancer rates have recently declined, from a high of 87 per 100,000 in 1984 to 80 in 1990. This decline in incidence, however, is limited to men under fifty-five years of age. This is the first such decrease in fifty years and corresponds to a substantial decrease in smoking patterns among men twenty years ago. Among women the story is different: Lung cancer incidence is still increasing steadily in women. No such decrease is expected for fifteen to twenty years because younger women are smoking more.

Breast-cancer incidence rates illustrate the effects of careful screening for the disease. The female breast cancer incidence rate increased from 85.2 per 100,000 in 1980 to 112.4 per 100,000 in 1987. In 1988, incidence rates actually decreased to 109.6 and further decreased in 1989 to 104.6. These specific trends in recent years appear to indicate a turnaround in breast cancer incidence rates. This trend supports the assumption that the increase during the 1980s was due to early detection resulting from the increased use of mammography.

Cancer of the prostate shows a consistent increase in the period covered. Doll and Peto believe this pattern to be the result of a "vigorous search for lumps" resulting in an

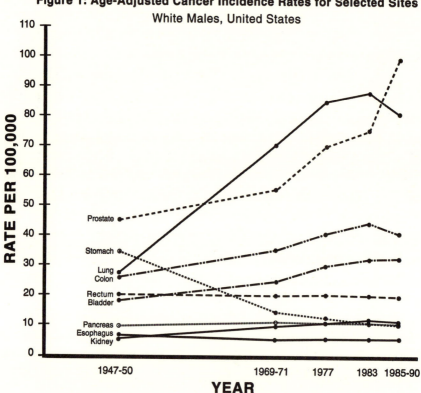

Figure 1: Age-Adjusted Cancer Incidence Rates for Selected Sites
White Males, United States

Source: Data from the NCI cancer incidence surveys (1947-50 and 1969-71) and SEER
(1977,1983, 1985-90) adjusted to the age distribution of the 1970 U.S. census population.

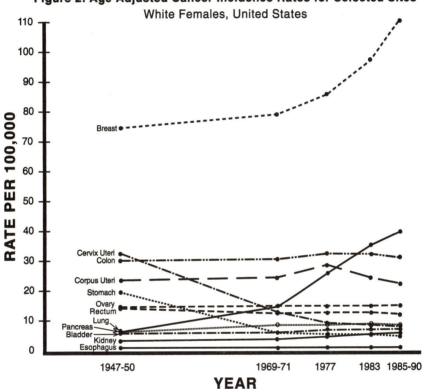

Figure 2: Age-Adjusted Cancer Incidence Rates for Selected Sites
White Females, United States

Source: Data from the NCI cancer incidence surveys (1947-50 and 1969-71) and SEER
(1977,1983, 1985-90) adjusted to the age distribution of the 1970 U.S. census population.

over-diagnosis of the disease in cases where it is associated with old age and is not life-threatening. Frequently, this apparent increase is detected as a result of biopsies for noncancerous conditions. However, the rise in incidence is mainly due to ultrasound examination and the routine use of the Prostate Specific Antigent (PSA) test. The average age at diagnosis for prostate cancer is about 73.

AGE-SPECIFIC INCIDENCE BAND

Thus far, we have used age-adjusted comparisons of incidence rates. Although these rates display useful trends, they do not give the full picture. Cancer becomes thirty times more common in women and one hundred times more common in men as age increases from twenty-five to seventy-five years. Changes in age-adjusted incidence in all ages reflect almost entirely changes in the older age groups. In order to assess the effect of recent changes in treatment and the prevalence of cancer-causing agents, trends in the younger age groups are particularly useful. The trends in young adults can reflect only relatively recent changes in the prevalence of carcinogenic agents and are not complicated by changes made in the distant past. Also young people tend to adopt new health habits more readily than older individuals.

Examination of the trends for various types of cancer at twenty to forty-four years of age reveals that increases in both sexes can be accounted for by the four types of cancer listed in Table 2.2. The biggest increase is seen in non-melanomatous skin cancer, which includes Kaposi's sarcoma. The second biggest increase is seen in non-Hodgkin's lymphoma. In both of these cases, the increases are far greater in men and can be attributed to the association

Table 2.2
Increases in Recorded Incidence of Cancer:
SEER Program, 1973-1977 to 1983-1987,
Ages 20-44 Years

	Incidence per 10,000 per year			
Type of Cancer	Men		Women	
	1973–1977	1983–1987 as % of 1973–1977	1973–1977	1983–1987 as % of 1973–1977
Testis	7.85	139*		
Melanoma	6.65	129*	8.28	131*
Non-Hodgkin's lymphoma	3.67	174*	2.72	116*
Skin, non-melanoma	0.37	2,246*	0.41	161*
Four types	18.54	185*	11.41	128*
Other cancers	42.83	96	96.18	99
All cancers	61.37	123	107.59	102

*p. 0.05
Source: R. Doll, "Progress Against Cancer: An Epidemiological Assessment,"
American Journal of Epidemiology 134, no. 7 (1 Oct 1991): 675–88.

of these diseases to the development of the acquired immuno-deficiency syndrome (AIDS). Thus, the increased incidence rates in this age group illustrate the introduction of a known cancer-inducing agent into the population—the human immunodeficiency virus (HIV).

The increases in melanoma are attributable to sun exposure in light-skinned populations. At the present moment, there is no explanation for the increase of testicular cancer seen in this younger age band.

Table 2.3 illustrates three forms of cancer that have decreased in incidence during the period covered. The reduction

Table 2.3
Reductions in Recorded Incidence of Cancer:
SEER Program, 1973-1977 to 1983-1987,
Ages 20-44 years

Type of Cancer	Incidence per 10,000 per year			
	Men		Women	
	1973–1977	1983–1987 as % of 1973–1977	1973–1977	1983–1987 as % of 1973–1977
Stomach	1.10	92	0.64	84
Lung	5.90	81*	4.22	91
Cervix			12.34	78*
Other cancers	30.69	101	27.13	102
Total	37.69	99	44.33	94

*p. 0.05

Source: R. Doll, "Progress Against Cancer: An Epidemiological Assessment," *American Journal of Epidemiology* 134, no. 7 (1 Oct 1991): 675-88.

in lung cancer incidence is due to the decreasing number of young men taking up smoking. The 22 percent decrease in cancer of the cervix in women may be attributed to the spread of cervical screening and early detection of the disease. The reason for the decrease in stomach cancer may be attributed to improved refrigeration, hygiene, and improved food preservation techniques. Again, the trends in this age band illustrate relatively recent changes in the health practices in the United States.

MORTALITY

Figures 3 and 4 present death rates for males and females respectively from 1930 until 1990 (the latest data available as of this writing). An important advantage of these data is the availability throughout the period.

The sharp increase in deaths from lung cancer is apparent, as is the sharp decrease in deaths due to stomach cancer. The other forms of cancer tend to show steady death rates, especially in recent years. There is no marked increase in mortality from prostate or breast cancer. This supports the argument that increases in incidence are largely artifactual. Death rates from stomach and cervical cancer also declined over the entire period, and those for colon and rectal cancer show a downward trend. Deaths from other cancers indicate a steady rate in recent years.

CANCER IN MINORITIES

Examination of current cancer patterns is an important step in addressing the issue of whether there is a cancer epidemic. For example, by comparing racial and ethnic groups at the same point in time we can specify which groups have high rates for specific cancers. This may indicate trends toward an epidemic. These comparisons have been examined for men and for women from the 1930s until 1990. Comparing groups at the same point in time allows us to eliminate biases in the data attributable to changes in recording procedures and diagnoses with the passage of time.

In 1994, of the expected 1,208,000 diagnosed cancers in the United States, about 120,000 will be among black Americans and 35,000 among other minority Americans.

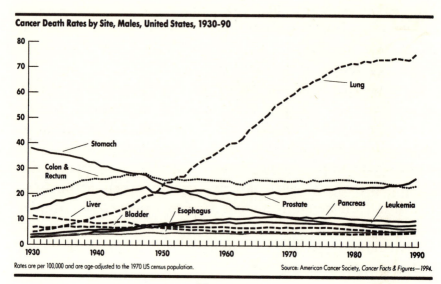

Cancer Death Rates by Site, Males, United States, 1930-90

Rates are per 100,000 and are age-adjusted to the 1970 US census population.   Source: American Cancer Society, *Cancer Facts & Figures—1994.*

Figure 3

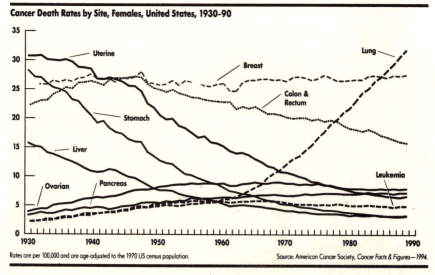

Cancer Death Rates by Site, Females, United States, 1930-90

Rates are per 100,000 and are age-adjusted to the 1970 US census population.   Source: American Cancer Society, *Cancer Facts & Figures—1994.*

Figure 4

In general, cancer incidence and mortality rates are higher for black Americans than for white Americans. In 1990, the incidence rates were 423 per 100,000 for blacks as opposed to 393 for whites. The mortality rates for the same year were 230 for blacks and 170 for whites. Black Americans have significantly higher incidence and mortality rates for the following forms of cancer: esophagus, uterine, cervix, stomach, liver, prostate, larynx, and multiple myeloma.

Incidence and mortality rates for other minority groups such as Hispanics are lower than those for white or black Americans. These comparisons confirm that a cancer epidemic exists among blacks in the United States. They further specify which types of cancer account for this epidemic. The specific causes for this epidemic may be the risks associated with various aspects of lifestyle and differences in access to health care.

ANOTHER WAY OF LOOKING AT CURRENT PATTERNS: GENDER

Another approach to current male-female cancer patterns is to look not at rates but at only the percentage distribution of deaths for the major forms of cancer among individuals who have the disease.

Each year, the American Cancer Society prepares estimates of the percentage distribution of cancer incidence and death by site and sex for the upcoming year. Since their projections for mortality tend to be much more accurate than those for incidence, only the mortality estimates are presented here (Figure 5).

The high percentage of expected death from lung cancer in men is readily apparent. Of the men expected to die from cancer in 1994, 33 percent were projected to die from lung

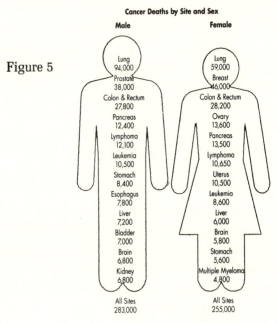

Cancer Deaths by Site and Sex

Figure 5

Source American Cancer Society Cancer Facts & Figures—1994

cancer. For women, the corresponding figure is 23 percent. The latter figure is of particular significance. Since 1987, lung cancer surpassed breast cancer as the major cause of cancer death in American women. Thus, by looking only at cancer victims we have again confirmed the presence of a lung cancer epidemic.

International

Sources of Data

The major source of data for international disease incidence and mortality rates is the World Health Organization (WHO), specificaily its affiliate the International Agency for Research on Cancer (IARC). Periodically, IARC publishes international incidence data, the latest volume being *Cancer Incidence in Five Continents,* volume 5 (1987). This volume contains data from 58 cancer registries, although it does not cover all countries on every continent. WHO also publishes updated data on mortality.

International Comparisons of Cancer Statistics

Comparisons of cancer incidence and mortality among countries presents many potential sources of error. Data for each country are subject to the kinds of error for incidence and mortality discussed earlier for the United States. Since the type of errors vary by country and registry, comparisons can serve to magnify errors.

Of particular importance is the fact that incidence data are usually based on a small number of registries in a particular country. The data fall into specifically identified regions, states, counties, and metropolitan areas, and it is unclear how representative these registries are for the total population of the country. In addition, the extent to which people use medical services (often varying according to age), the availability and affordability of these services, the level of diagnostic ability, and the quality of data in the registry— compliance in reporting, careful checks, and "cleaning" of the data—may all differ by registry and county. For these reasons, we limit our analysis to a comparison of mortality data.

A major problem with mortality rates is that the level of technology used in diagnosis and the medical treatment given to the patient can affect lifespan. Therefore, a high or low mortality rate may not truly reflect the cancer mortality, but rather the influence of the level of diagnosis and treatment.

Because of these limitations we will primarily rely on the international data to help confirm the epidemic of lung cancer already found in the time comparisons. Of course, there is also the possibility that the U.S. data for a particular site will not reveal an epidemic when in fact international comparisons do. Because of the serious limitations of international data, evaluation of these findings is beyond the scope of this report.

Internationally compared cancer incidence and mortality data are age-standardized to a world standard population. Sometimes different world standard populations are used for different continents. However, despite this precaution the influence of age can exert an effect on the data through such processes as differential use of diagnostic and treatment facilities by various age groups.

Mortality rates are available for forty-six countries. Table 2.4 presents the U.S. world standardized rate and rank for all sites combined for eight major cancers. The overall rates and ranks indicate no evidence for a cancer epidemic for either sex. While the mortality data are consistent with an epidemic of lung cancer for both sexes, there is nonetheless no conclusive evidence of an overall cancer epidemic in the United States.

Hysterical Media Perceptions of a "Cancer Epidemic"

"So, I guess this doesn't make much difference," sighed an acquaintance of mine at the pool club the other day. "What

Table 2.4
U.S. Mortality Rate per 100,000 and
Rank Among 50 Countries for Cancer,
Selected Sites by Sex, 1986-88*

	Male		Female	
	Rate	Rank	Rate	Rank
All Sites	163.2	24	109.7	17
Oral	3.8	30	1.4	13
Colon & Rectum	17.2	22	12.0	21
Lung	56.9	12	22.7	4
Breast			22.4	16
Uterus				
Cervix			2.7	37
Other			2.7	33
Stomach	5.3	49	2.3	49
Prostate	15.7	22		
Leukemia	6.3	10	3.8	14

*Age-adjusted death rates per 100,000 population. Rates are adjusted to the WHO world standard population.
Source: World Health Statistics Annuals 1987–1990.

do you mean?" I wondered as we began our daily exercise routine. "We baby boomers—no matter how healthy we try to be—are doomed. We're going to get cancer anyway—I heard it on the news this week."

My colleague in the pursuit of good health was referring to recent press accounts claiming that new data now indicate an increased cancer rate among those of us born during the 1940s—even if we do not smoke cigarettes. The various media reports refer to a recent article published by the prestigious *Journal of the American Medical Association* (*JAMA*) and written by a team of government scientists headed by Dr.

Devra Lee Davis. The media coverage generated by this report was indeed alarming, especially if one reviews some of these headlines: "Cancer Risk Up Sharply In This Era" proclaimed the *Washington Post;* "Study Finds Increase In Cancer Risk For White Baby Boomers" concurred *The Seattle Times.* The reports all stated that environmental, non-tobacco-related factors are the underlying cause for this apparent "dramatic increase." The Clinton administration is already citing these new data to bolster its regulatory assault on "carcinogens," particularly the much-maligned agricultural chemicals—e.g., pesticides.

When I read the issue of *JAMA* which published this article, I found that the media (a) apparently limited itself to reporting only on the article itself, not the accompanying editorial written by Dr. Anthony B. Miller which largely dismissed the findings, and (b) did not share with consumers some of the obvious shortcomings of the *JAMA* piece— limitations which are critical in interpreting its conclusions. We need to examine the limitations of the *JAMA* article, as well as the political movement behind the search for hypothetical environmental causes of cancer.

FLAWS IN STUDY DESIGN

The most significant problem with the *JAMA* article is the fact that Dr. Davis and her colleagues attempted to understate the effects of tobacco in cancer causation. These authors estimate that 30 percent of cancers are tobacco-related, yet the prevailing view is that more than 40 percent of all cancer cases (excluding superficial skin cancers) in the 1990s are caused by tobacco. This is particularly true in the baby-boom cohort, the group that is of concern to Dr. Davis and her colleagues, because of the dramatic increase in female smoking after 1945. This underestimation of the effects of tobacco leaves room for subsequent speculation that cancer must be caused by unseen "environmental causes."

The authors also manipulate data from the National Cancer Institute by attempting to separate cigarette-caused cancers from those not linked with smoking. This is a critically important division because of the enormous contribution of tobacco use to cancer frequency in the decades after 1940. Thus, while the authors limited the category "cigarette-related cancers" to the traditional sites (lung, oral cavity, esophagus), epidemiologists now attribute a significant portion of cancer at other sites, including pancreas, kidney, bladder, and cervix, to cigarette smoking. Most recently, a study published in the *Journal of the National Cancer Institute* (*JNCI*) linked smoking to the causation of colon cancer—a previously unrecognized connection. The *JNCI* study found that smoking doubled the risk of developing colon cancer thirty-five years after a person became addicted to cigarettes. The evidence seems to indicate that the artificial categories created by the authors are indeed meaningless—few cancer sites could truly be excluded from the "cigarette-related cancers" category. If the authors had expanded their definition of cigarette-related cancer, the conclusions of the article would have changed significantly.

INCONSISTENT ANALYSES

Davis and her co-authors make clear that their analysis of cancer data relates mainly to *incidence*. The distinction between incidence and mortality may, however, be lost on most lay readers. Mortality, as the term suggests, refers to deaths from cancer. Incidence refers to the number of new cases diagnosed. Thus, any increased use of modern medical technology—like the Pap smear for cervical cancer, PSA for prostate cancer, and mammograms for breast cancer—could dramatically increase incidence, without a similar increase in mortality. Cancer of the breast and prostate both illustrate this point—both have increased in incidence, without a correspondingly large change in mortality. Indeed, it could be argued that increasing incidence of many cancers is good news in that it is a sign of finding cancers early and allowing the type of intervention that potentially saves lives.

As the title of the *JAMA* article suggests, the authors wish to portray the data as the "Good News and Bad News" of causes of death in the United States. Indeed, one cannot evaluate the frequency of one major disease, like cancer, without considering trends in "competing" causes of illness and death. In fact, recent studies indicate that 30 percent of the increase in cancer mortality between 1973 and 1987 was due to competing risks. If, as the data suggests, the United States has experienced a major decline in mortality due to cardiovascular disease, other causes of death should increase proportionally. A cure for heart disease would make the cancer incidence and mortality rate *soar*. Humans remain mortal. Something has to be the leading cause of death!

Dr. Davis and her colleagues did not consider an additional "risk" factor for cancer—AIDS, with its associated decrease in immunity which frequently leads to death by cancer. Such prominent epidemiolgists as Sir Richard Doll stress the fact that in order to assess the effect of recent changes in treatment and the prevalence of cancer-causing agents, trends seen in younger age groups are particularly useful. The trends in young adults reflect only relatively recent changes in the prevalence of carcinogenic agents and are not complicated by exposures in the distant past. The authors neglected to analyze the effects of such proven "environmental factors" as the introduction of the human immunodeficiency virus (HIV) on cancer incidence, particularly in these important younger age groups. Instead, they focused their discussion on baby boomers and the elderly.

Indeed, cancer incidence for forms of cancer related to AIDS has increased in these younger age groups (20–44 years of age). The biggest increase is seen in non-melanomatous skin cancer, which includes Kaposi's sarcoma. The second biggest increase is seen in non-Hodgkin's lymphoma. In both cases, the increases are far greater in men. Thus, the increased incidence rates for cancer in this age group illustrate the introduction of a known cancers-promoting agent into the population—HIV—and do not support the conclusion of "unseen environmental hazards" as the authors suggest.

UNSUBSTANTIATED CONCLUSIONS AND THEIR EFFECTS

Scientists count among their recreational activities "lemon squeeze" sessions where they pick apart the published work of colleagues, pointing to specific omissions or shortcomings. This is all fair sport at academic seminars, and scientists understand that one study does not a conclusion make. Journals such as *JAMA* have no qualms about publishing studies with which many editors might disagree because they know there will be in-context dialogue after publication to resolve differences. (In this instance, *JAMA* began this discussion by publishing its critical dialogue in the same issue.) The problem here then was not the Davis article itself, but the fact that it was plucked out of context and reported uncritically by the press.

What was unusual about the article, however, was that the authors ventured beyond their tenuous conclusions that there was a cancer "epidemic" to offer a possible cause: environmental chemicals, particularly pesticides. Why did they point to agricultural chemicals? Because, they said, there was epidemiological data that farmers had an increased risk of cancer and they thought that occupational risk might carry over to consumers who eat the food farmers produce. Here, then, is a major flaw in the *JAMA* piece: if indeed farmers do have an increased risk (yet unproven) related to their use of chemicals on the farm, what possible relevance would that have to us and our occasional parts per billion (or less) exposure to pesticide residues in food? Extrapolating from a high-dose occupational exposure to a minuscule intermittent general exposure would be like concluding that those of us who have an annual x-ray are at risk just because radiologists, who years ago practiced their specialty daily, without protection, had a higher cancer risk.

Out of all the possible reasons to speculate on why nonsmoking baby boomers might have an allegedly higher cancer risk, why zoom in on pesticides? Why not speculate instead that it was a myriad of other reasons—such as marijuana use—or the increased consumption of vegetables and fruits (with their naturally occurring carcinogens) that caused the alleged increase?

The answers to the above questions become clear when one investigates the political movement behind this search for hypothetical "environmental risks." Dr. Davis is considered by many to be a "maverick" in this political movement. She is among a group of scientists proposing that "synthetic chemicals are permeating the environment" and that mimicking hormones, such as estrogen, possibly cause cancer. In fact, the media coverage generated by this article is strangely reminiscent of a similar *Journal of the National Cancer Institute* (*JNCI*) study published last year which received considerable attention. The study, titled "Blood Levels of Organochlorine Residues and Risk of Breast Cancer," was designed to determine whether DDT and PCBs are associated with increased breast cancer risk in women. The principal investigators were Dr. Mary S. Wolff and her colleagues at the Mount Sinai Medical School. According to the researchers, their data showed a "fourfold increase in the relative risk of breast cancer for an elevation of serum DDE [a by-product of DDT found in the body]." No similar association could be made for PCBs.

The findings of this study, like the recent *JAMA* article, were overemphasized by the media. The media and environmental groups have used the results of the Wolff study— a small, preliminary investigation—as evidence of a definitive link between organochlorine pesticides and cancer. A series of articles appeared in major newspapers across the country with such titles as "First DDT Link to Breast Cancer Reported." An accompanying editorial, written by David J. Hunter and Karl T. Kelsey, went so far as to state that the "findings of Wolff *et al.* may have *extraordinary global implications* for the prevention of breast cancer" and "their study should serve as a *wake-up call* for further urgent research." (emphasis added)

The Wolff study, like the Davis article, raises more questions than it answers. For example, DDT was banned in the United States in 1972, but its use worldwide is greater today than it was then. Is one of the "global implications" of Wolff's paper that DDT should be banned worldwide? (Discontinuing the use of DDT could lead to a dramatic increase in insect-borne disease.) Why investigate DDT exposure in New York? DDT was "overused" primarily in the Southern United States. Is the increased incidence of breast cancer in Long Island related to some "unseen" over-exposure to the chemical? When was this cohort of women exposed? Did the exposure occur in New York? (No data is provided in the Wolff article to suggest when and where the exposure to DDT occurred.) Many critics question the validity of the Wolff data because the study did not control for dietary fat intake. Would controlling for such variables greatly alter the results of the Wolff study?

The studies conducted by Drs. Wolff and Davis add fuel to the fire of the politicized scientific debate. What worried baby boomers—and the environmental activists now pressuring the Administration to "do something" to reduce our cancer risk—need to keep in mind is that the science of cancer epidemiology still points to lifestyle factors (cigarette smoking, excessive sun exposure), not environ-mental chemicals, as the primary, controllable causes of cancer. As Dr. Clark Heath, vice president for epidemiology and statistics at the American Cancer Society stated in recent media reports: "I don't think the study changes our per-spective on . . . what causes cancer."

Before we begin redirecting funds from such valuable pursuits as searches for effective treatments, policy makers need to decide if searching for "toxic phantoms" will be a fruitful endeavor or yet another unnecessary burden on our public health research budget. We need to prevent a dis-proportionate amount of research dollars from going into relatively low priority fields at the expense of programs that directly benefit the cancer patient. We cannot guide public policy by the uncritical, out-of-context reporting of scientific data by the media. Such action would be hazardous to the health of all of us.

3

Tobacco

Cigarettes are killers that travel in packs.

—Mary S. Ott

Tobacco, Pro and Con

A custom loathsome to the eye, hateful to the Nose, harmful to the brain, dangerous to the Lungs, and in the black stinking fume thereof nearest resembling the horrible Stigian smoke of the pit that is bottomless ... for it is a stinking loathsome thing and so is hell. . . . If I were to invite the devil to dinner, he should have three dishes: first a pig, second a pull and a ling of mustard, and a pipe of tobacco.

In 1604, King James I of England used these words to condemn the use of tobacco in no uncertain terms. He wished that Sir Francis Drake and Sir Walter Raleigh had never introduced the habit in the 1580s. He probably rued the day that Columbus became so enthralled with the natives of San Salvador, who blew great clouds of smoke from their nostrils that, he brought tobacco back with him and started popularizing tobacco use in Spain, France, and England.

Tobacco has been a controversial topic among physicians and laypeople for centuries. While King James and others were condemning it, placing heavy taxes on it, and threatening punishments which included nose amputation, others were proclaiming its magical medical properties. "Herba Panacea" was recommended to cure cancer, epilepsy, arthritis, and "other diseases of the Lungs and Inward Parties." Real aficionados claimed, strangely enough, "It maketh the voice clear. . . . It maketh the breath sweet."

Health warnings and predictions of moral decline had little effect on the growing popularity of tobacco use—in pipes, as snuff, and for chewing. Although for each tobacco enthusiast there was an equally emphatic nonuser who abhorred the stuff, in the first 250 years after the tobacco plant was brought from the New World there were no documented reports that tobacco was linked to cancer. There were, of course, individual clinical opinions expressed that tobacco was harmful to health. For example, in the late 1600s, a Dr. Evard of London wrote that "tobacco causes vomit and is an enemy of the stomach." However, cancer was not mentioned as the result of smoking any more often than was any other illness.

In 1761, an English physician made the first clinical report documenting that tobacco use led to cancer. In that year Dr. John Hill presented his *Cautions Against the Immoderate Use of Snuff.* He told of two cases of nasal cancer, both victims with "polypusses" that he thought were malignant. He described the first case in his document:

This unfortunate gentleman, after a long and immoderate use of Snuff, perceived that he breathed with difficulty through one of his nostrils; the complaint gradually increased, 'til he perceived a swelling within. . . . It grew slowly, 'til in the end, it filled up that whole nostril, and swelled the nose so as to obstruct the breathing . . . he found it necessary to then apply for assistance. The swelling was quite black and it adhered by a broad base, so that it was impossible to attempt the getting it away . . . and the consequence was a discharge of a thin sharp tumor with dreadful pain, and all the frightful symptoms of cancer . . . and he seemed without hope when I last saw him.

His second description of a victim of snuff:

The person was a lady of a sober and virtuous life. . . . She had long been accustomed to Snuff and took it in a very great quantity. . . . She felt a strange soreness in the upper part of her nostril. . . . After a little time, came on a discharge of a very offensive matter; not in any quantity but of an intolerable smell, and was more so to her, as she was naturally a person of great delicacy. The discharge increased, and it soon became necessary for her to leave off Snuff. A surgeon was employed, but to very little purpose.

So in 1761, Dr. Hill was describing malignancies. He clearly blamed tobacco, in the form of snuff. According to modern evidence, he was probably right—now we see an increase in oral cancers among snuff-dippers, since the fashion has changed from putting snuff up the nose to somewhere in the mouth (usually between the lips and the teeth).

Dr. Hill's observations, however, were never given much thought. People kept on smoking, sniffing, and chewing.

Throughout the 1800s other reports occasionally suggested that tobacco use was associated with cancer. (Until this century tobacco use included only pipes, cigars, chewing tobacco, and snuff. Cigarettes were not "invented" until relatively later.) In 1849, a Boston surgeon wrote that "for more than twenty years back I have been in the habit of inquiring of patients who come to me with cancers . . . of the gums . . . tongue and lips . . . whether they use tobacco. . . . When, as is usually the case, one side of the tongue is affected with ulcerated cancer, the tobacco has been habitually retained in contact with that part." The same year Dr. John Shew published his book *Tobacco: Its History, Nature, and Effects on the Body and Mind,* which asked: "I believe cancers . . . and tumors in and about the mouth will be found much more common among men than women. Since the former use tobacco much more generally than the latter, may not this be the cause?"

In 1859, a French doctor named Bouisson presented his study of sixty-eight patients who had cancer of the oral cavity. The majority (two-thirds) of them had cancer of the lip, and the others had various others of the mouth, tongue, tonsil, inside of the cheek, and gums. Sixty-six of the patients smoked tobacco and one chewed tobacco. Bouisson also noted that the cancers most often occurred at the spot where the pipe or cigar was held against the oral area.

The Invention—the Cigarette

All the earlier reports were limited to tobacco chewers and sniffers, and pipe and cigar smokers. Just as evidence was building that these forms of tobacco were related to cancer, cigarettes were introduced to Britain by the troops that had fought in the Crimean War.

The first cigarettes were makeshift, rolled by hand by the user out of loose tobacco. They were not very popular for several reasons. First, they took so long to make properly that they were available only in limited quantities (they were "just too much trouble"). Second, when compared to pipes and cigars, cigarettes seemed effeminate. "Tell me what you smoke and I'll tell you who you are," was the slogan of the day. Real men didn't want to smoke pretty "little cigars" wrapped in white paper.

The situation changed when the automatic cigarette rolling machine was invented in the 1870s. By 1885, cigarettes became available and cheap, and were accepted in European and American society.

The year 1885 also marked the death of General Ulysses S. Grant, a cigar smoker, from throat cancer. In the public mind, his cigar smoking was associated with his military prowess. One of his favorite gifts from admirers after his military defeat of the South in the Civil War was a collection of some 11,000 cigars. Medical reports of the last days before his death indicate that his pain was so great he had to sleep sitting up to relieve the pressure and pain of his spreading cancer.

By 1900, cigarettes had established popularity in the United States. They not only were readily available, but they were so mild that the smoke could be inhaled into the lungs (which cruder tobacco products like cigars and pipe tobacco could not). They also fit in to the fast-paced American lifestyle that was developing. Cigars and pipes were for men of leisure, to be savored after dinner with a snifter of brandy. Cigarettes were smaller, easier to carry around, and smoked rapidly—just the thing for the busy man on the move.

As cigarette smoking became more popular before World War I, complaints from antitobacco leagues grew. Cigarettes were again called "inventions of the devil," "likely to ruin one's morals," and "coffin nails"—threats to health. The charges made against smoking were carried in books with titles like *The Use of Tobacco vs. Purity, Chastity and Good Health*. And the claims of the antitobacconists were so wrapped up in moral and ethical aspects of questions that the possible health effects were ignored.

The debate ran on—every time someone suggested prohibiting smoking, someone else countered that the habit was beneficial. In 1906, a doctor lamented that modern women were drinking too much tea and advised that they take up smoking, as nicotine would counteract the stimulant in tea and thus prevent heart attacks. In 1911, when a French physician was asked about cancer that had occurred in smokers, he answered that the cancers could well have occurred anyway, and that the smoking may have just determined the location. In 1918, the *New York Times* ran the headlines "surgeons laud cigarettes" and a story that recommended servicemen be given a full supply of them as "the effect of the cigarette is wonderful."

In 1911, a new job was established, that of "cigarette sampler." As the job description read, "all he has to do is give away an occasional pack with tact and discretion." The industry was on its way, selling more and more of its product and successfully soliciting scores of new customers.

There seemed to be reason for concern—this was, after all, the first time in history that men (and a few sly women) were drawing hot cigarette smoke directly into their lungs. But no one thought of lung cancer.

In 1912, a Dr. I. Adler wrote about disease patterns in the United States: "There is nearly complete consensus of opinion that primary malignant neoplasms of the lung are among the rarest forms of disease." Most medical students training at that time never saw a case of lung cancer.

Cigarette sales increased steadily to 1918, but World War I gave them an extra push, as tobacco was used to assuage the troops. General Pershing, Commander-in-Chief of the American Troops in France, once cabled Washington saying, "Tobacco is as indispensable as the daily ration; we must have thousands of tons of it without delay." After the war, cigarettes became even more popular. An article in the *New York Times* said, "Tobacco affords true enjoyment; it helps our organism over many difficulties and over many cares and hardships leading to a depressed state. It satisfies thirst and hunger, as we learned during the war."

The years between 1920 and 1940 were the heyday of smoking. Dr. John Harvey Kellogg, in his book *Tobaccoism: How Tobacco Kills* (1922), accused smoking of causing cancers of the lip, throat, and mouth, but he was not taken seriously. Even outspoken advocates of the Anti-tobacco League, which had all the vim and vigor of the Women's Christian Temperance Union prior to prohibition (their efforts led to the passing of the 23rd Amendment), had little effect. Miss Lucy Page Gaston, leader of the Anti-tobacco League, wrote to President Harding, begging him not to smoke. Jovial cigarette lovers responded by organizing a "cigarettes for Harding" campaign. Five years later, President Coolidge and Vice President Dawes were also asked not to smoke. But they kept on puffing away.

During Prohibition, cigarettes offered a legal form of personal comfort (although it never entirely took the place of demon rum).

Testimonials appeared frequently in the *Times:* "Smoked Seventy Years, Now Celebrating his Hundredth Birthday"; "Doctor scoffs at charges that cigarettes interfere with health"; "Smoking promotes health, MDs say. It increases the flow of gastric juices and contributes to evenness of temper." In October 1926, a front-page story told of the findings of a Johns Hopkins professor who decided that "smoking makes men more dependable," since it was thought to act as a sedative. True, he said, "smoking does increase blood pressure slightly, but so does telling a good joke." According to him, smoking was good for you, and people believed him.

Some smokers were undoubtedly amused by a 1929 *Times* article, "Three year old Boy is Regular Smoker." Maurice St. Pierre of Waterbury, Connecticut, was said to have smoked two cigars daily, ten pipesful of tobacco, and a pack of cigarettes. The story added that he lit his own, and had taken up the habit at the age of one-and-a-half.

By 1935, nearly everyone smoked. The radio ads constantly sang cigarettes' praises, touting their great range of sizes and brands. The Prince of Wales even came up with a half-size cigarette he claimed was ideal for puffing between dances.

Prestigious doctors testified in advertisements that cigarettes were kind to the throat, and opera singers claimed, "We protect our voices with Lucky Strikes." Models dressed in Lucky Strike green danced up and down New York City's

Fifth Avenue smoking cigarettes. Then came what may have been one of the most successful ad campaigns in history— "Reach for a Lucky instead of a Sweet." Chocolate sales declined and industry spokesmen claimed that "the cigarette is a deadly enemy of chocolate." Weight-watching women became interested in cigarettes (but, thankfully, *Good Housekeeping* magazine protested, "We're just old-fashioned enough to wish that women would not smoke."), just as the taboo on female smoking began to lift. In 1934, Mrs. Franklin Roosevelt became the first (known) lady to smoke in public.

By 1935, although the habit was still more popular with men, female smoking was picking up momentum. Sixty-six percent of the male population and 26 percent of the female population under the age of forty smoked cigarettes. In contrast, smoking was almost unheard of at the beginning of the twentieth century.

The Case Against Smoking Develops

Unbeknownst to the ever-growing smoking public, an impressive amount of speculation along with hard scientific evidence linked smoking with disease beginning in the 1920s. All of it was ignored by the tobacco companies, who continued to promote their deadly products with reckless abandon.

In the 1920s, a University of Minnesota pathologist, Dr. Moses Barron, noticed an unusually high occurrence of lung cancer, a relatively rare disease for the time. His ensuing investigation confirmed a dramatic increase in lung cancer rates during the twenty-two-year period from 1899 to 1921.

In a July 30, 1927, letter to the editor of *Lancet*, Dr. Frank E. Tylecote wrote:

As a clinician, I have remarks to make: (1) It might be assumed that the incidence of lung cancer is limited mainly to the working class. This is by no means the case; in Manchester we have lost several well-known public men from this disease in recent years. (2) I have no statistics with regard to tobacco, but I think that in almost every case I have seen and know of the patient has been a regular smoker, generally of cigarettes.

Also around 1930, a German scientist named Lickint reported that 3400 out of 4000 bronchial cancer patients were men. He thought that the sex difference could be explained by smoking habits. And he went even further. Not only did he postulate that smoking increased the risk of getting lung cancer, but he thought that the by-products of inhaled cigarette smoke might filter through to the bladder and remain there, to cause cancer (and his idea, the Lickint Hypothesis, was confirmed some thirty-five years later). In March of 1930, the *Journal of the American Medical Association* (*JAMA*) carried his findings, but no one paid much attention to them. In fact, after careful consideration, in November 1933 *JAMA* carried its first cigarette advertisement (Chesterfields), a practice that was to continue for twenty years.

In a 1931 volume of the *Annals of Surgery,* Dr. Frederick Hoffman commented on his own clinical experience that "smoking habits unquestionably increase the liability to cancer of the mouth, the throat, the esophagus, the larynx, and the lungs." No one paid much attention to his findings either.

In 1939, Dr. Phillip Matz recalled that lung cancer was practically unheard of in 1912, and wondered why his autopsy records at the Veterans Hospital in Washington showed that deaths from lung cancer had increased 121 percent from 1931 to 1937. In comparison, other cancers had increased by only 28 percent.

Also in 1939, Dr. F. Mueller reported in Germany's chief cancer journal (*Zeitschrift für Krebsforschung*) that eighty-three out of eighty-six lung cancer patients smoked. Both physicians and laymen laughed at his reports. The over-whelming response was that something besides cigarettes was responsible for the noted increase in lung cancer. Perhaps, some reckoned, there wasn't even a real increase. Rather, techniques had improved so much since 1900 that doctors could now better diagnose the disease (an "increase in reporting"). Or, if there really was an increase in lung cancer rates, perhaps it was due to industrialization, tarred roads, or delayed complications of the devastating 1918 influenza epidemic. Certainly cigarettes could not be implicated, not when they offered so much pleasure to so many Americans.

In February of 1936, Dr. Aaron Arkin and Dr. David Wagner of the University of Chicago publicized their concern about the increase in lung cancer cases. "Ninety percent of all our patients were chronic smokers, and we believe that the inhalation of tobacco smoke may be an important factor in producing chronic irritation." At the International Cancer Congress in 1939, Dr. Alton Ochsner, a surgeon from New Orleans and noted heart surgeon Dr. Michael DeBakey declared: "It's our conviction that the increase in pulmonary carcinoma is due largely to the increase in smoking, particularly cigarette smoking, which is universally associated with inhalation."

By today's standards, the medical evidence gathered against cigarettes would surely be enough to stimulate a thorough investigation of the matter and definitely elicit coverage in the popular press. But, unfortunately, this was not the case in the 1930s. The large metropolitan newspapers were fattening on tobacco advertising and the last thing they wanted to print was bad news about one of their best clients. And, due to the success of the cigarette advertising campaigns, the majority of American men, including physicians and scientists who were the first to be made aware of the alarming new data, were smokers themselves. They thus found it rather hard to admit that a habit to which they had become both psychologically and physiologically addicted was a major threat to their health and lives, so they resorted to denial of the obvious facts. And the advertising of cigarettes in *JAMA* continued. "More Doctors Smoke Camels," "The Thoughtful Physician Sends Cigarettes to His Friends and Patients Overseas."

The one exception to the general silence on the tobacco-health issue was a study done by Dr. Raymond Pearl of Johns Hopkins appearing in *Science* in 1938. He found that 54 percent of 100,000 heavy smokers (defined as those who smoked ten or more cigarettes a day) died before the age of fifty. In contrast, just 43 percent of 100,000 nonsmokers died before the age of fifty. He concluded that "smoking is associated with a definite impairment of longevity." While it was only a vague conclusion, it was certainly a start, and it did make the headlines. Pearl, who was a biostatistician, was roundly criticized by the medical press, which proclaimed, "Extensive scientific studies have proved that smoking in moderation by those for whom tobacco is not especially contra-indicated does not appreciably shorten life." A 1948 *JAMA* editorial stated that "in all probability, more can be said in behalf of smoking as a form of escape from tension than against it."

The Ax Is Raised

During the same year, Dr. Evarts Graham and Ernst Wynder, a student at the Washington University School of Medicine, puzzled over the phenomenal rise in lung cancer deaths. Wynder hypothesized that there was probably an important correlation between the rise in cigarette use and lung cancer, but Dr. Graham was not convinced. He pointed out that there was also a correlation between increasing lung cancer rates and sales of nylon stockings.

Nevertheless, the two of them looked into the problem. Graham had a personal interest in the subject: in 1933 he had become the first physician to successfully remove a cancerous human lung (from a Pittsburgh obstetrician). He had first-hand clinical evidence of what people were saying might be the consequence of cigarette smoking. Perhaps he was interested in the hypothesis because he also was a smoker.

In 1949, Graham and Wynder began a study of 684 lung cancer patients, almost all male, at Washington University School Of Medicine in St. Louis. They found that 94 percent smoked cigarettes, around 3 percent smoked cigars, and some 3 percent smoked pipes. A few were nonsmokers or very light smokers.

Perhaps, they questioned, these results showed up because almost everyone smoked. To answer this question, the researchers looked at a group of control hospital patients, that is, hospitalized patients without lung cancer. Heavy and chain smoking was twice as common among lung cancer patients as compared to controls. In addition, nearly 15 percent of controls were nonsmokers.

Dr. Graham and soon-to-be Dr. Wynder reported their

results in the May 1950 issue of *JAMA*. "Extensive and prolonged use of tobacco, especially cigarettes, seems to be an important factor in the inducement of bronchogenic carcinoma."

In Great Britain, similar studies were taking place. In September 1950, the *British Medical Journal* carried an article entitled "Smoking and Carcinoma of the Lung," by Drs. Richard Doll and A. Bradford Hill. These researchers explained that they were puzzled by the huge increase in deaths due to lung cancer. They noted that the changing incidence in this form of death was the most dramatic ever recorded by England's Registrar General. In the twenty-five years between 1922 and 1947, the yearly number of lung-cancer deaths increased fifteenfold.

To the question "Why?" Doll and Hill had two possible answers: (1) the effects of air pollution from industry, automobile exhaust fumes, dust from tarred roads and coal fired, or (2) tobacco smoking.

Twenty hospitals in London participated in their ensuing study, notifying Doll and Hill of all patients admitted with the diagnosis of lung carcinoma. These patients and a similar number of controls were interviewed, and the results were parallel to those found by the American researchers just a few months before. For men, less than 0.3 percent of lung cancer patients were nonsmokers, compared with 4 percent of those without lung cancer.

It may seem confusing that these results are significant when it seems that almost everyone smoked. From a statistical point of view, though, the difference between 0.3 and 4 percent nonsmokers in the cases and control groups, respectively, is highly significant.

Medical researchers became more interested in cigarettes'

cancer-producing potential after these reports emerged. And the public press also became interested. In 1950, *Reader's Digest* ran an article called "How Harmful Are Cigarettes?" focusing on the two major preliminary reports and raising questions on the safety of smoking. This article was their first in a long line of attempts to notify the public of smoking's dangers. In contrast, a 1950 issue of *Coronet* featured an article, "The Facts About Cigarettes and Your Health," proclaiming the whole connection between smoking and lung cancer a hoax. The authors of this latter piece had "examined some fifty pounds of medical books and journals" to come to their conclusions, and ended by comparing the "cigarette-cancer hoax" to Orson Welles' "War of the Worlds" broadcast.

Doll and Hill continued to gather more information on lung cancer victims. In 1952, they informed the *British Medical Journal* of a definite association between cigarette smoking and lung cancer. The same year *Reader's Digest* ran an article called "Cancer by the Carton." The author told readers that at the time he began writing the piece he had been a two-pack-a-day smoker, but by the time he finished it he was sufficiently worried to limit himself to ten cigarettes a day.

Critics argued that more proof was needed, saying that the statistical observation that lung cancer patients are more likely to be smokers than people without lung cancer was not enough. What we needed, they felt, was a long-term study that followed a group of healthy smokers to see how many developed lung cancer.

The Ax Falls

Doll and Hill gathered information from forty thousand physicians, age thirty-five and older, including whether or not they smoked. After the questionnaires were returned, they kept track of all of the participants for four and a half years, obtaining death certificates on all who died. The results of their long-term study was that "mild smokers are seven times as likely to die of lung cancer as non-smokers; moderate smokers are twelve times as likely to die of lung cancer as non-smokers; immoderate smokers are twenty-four times as likely to die of lung cancer than non-smokers."

Herein was the first "proof" and more soon followed. In the United States Drs. E. Cuyler Hammond and Daniel Horn were conducting an even more extensive study for the American Cancer Society. They used 22,000 volunteers to interview over 187,000 men in nine states about their smoking habits. Interviewees were then followed for forty-four months.

Dr. Hammond smoked four packs a day, and Dr. Horn smoked one pack a day. As the last IBM card flipped out of the sorter, both of them switched to pipes. They were convinced. The total death rate from all causes combined was far higher in cigarette smokers than it was among non-smokers or cigar or pipe smokers. The death rate increased directly in proportion to the number of cigarettes smoked.

Studies went on through the 1950s and the 1960s, and the results were always the same. Cigarette smoking was harmful to health. In desperation, smokers suggested that perhaps it was not cigarette smoke causing the damage, but some other factor that cigarette smokers happened to have in common. A computer analysis looked at height, race, nativity, occupation, education, alcohol consumption, and other criteria and confirmed that the only difference between lung cancer victims and those without lung cancer was cigarette smoking.

The tide turned in 1957. On June 5, the *New York Times* carried a front-page story announcing "Cigarette Smoking Linked to Cancer in High Degree."

Sadly enough, Dr. Evarts Graham, one of the early researchers on the subject of smoking and lung cancer, never lived long enough to read that headline. Although he had given up smoking for good in 1953, for him it was too late. The late Dr. Alton Ochsner described the saddest letter he ever got from anyone was the one he received from Graham two weeks before he died. In it he said, "Because of our long friendship, you will be interested in knowing that they found that I have cancer in both my lungs. As you know, I stopped smoking several years ago but after having smoked as much as I did for so many years, too much damage has been done."

On June 1, 1961, the American Cancer Society, the American Heart Association, the American Public Health Association and the National Tuberculosis Association wrote a joint letter to President Kennedy emphasizing some of the dangers of cigarette smoking. They also pointed out the future consequences in terms of loss of life and economic productivity "unless appropriate health measure are taken." On June 7, The Surgeon General announced that a committee had been established to look into the subject as the health organizations had requested. On January 11, 1964, the committee made its final report:

Cigarette smoking is a health hazard of sufficient importance in the United States to warrant remedial action. . . .

Cigarette smoking is causally related to lung cancer in men; the magnitude of the effect of cigarette smoking far outweighs other factors. The data for women, although less extensive, point in the same direction.

Are We Sure That Cigarettes Cause Cancer?

"It would be hard to find another subject so thoroughly and extensively investigated during the last 25 years," said Dr. E. Cuyler Hammond of the American Cancer Society. *More than 60,000 scientific studies have consistently demonstrated that cigarettes are a major cause of cancer and other diseases. Not one legitimate major medical or scientific organization in the world denies that smoking is responsible for serious disease and premature death.*

If we had just a fraction of the evidence implicating cigarettes for other suspected carcinogens, there would be no controversy about them at all. If it had been any other substance, too, perhaps it might have been outlawed.

But it was not any other substance. Instead, it was tobacco, a product that has a substantial hold on a significant part of the world's population, including doctors. It also has tremendous monetary importance for U.S. Agribusiness, as tobacco is a cash crop in sixteen states.

So, the tobacco industry found a fairly receptive audience when it began its campaign to convince the public that there was still some doubt over the harmfulness of cigarettes. By means of news conferences, publications that counter specific charges against cigarettes, and with the help of something they call the Tobacco Action Network (TAN), the industry has been able to keep the cigarette "controversy" alive to this very day. The industry is constantly on the defense, asserting over and over again that the case against cigarettes remains "unproven." Unfortunately, for the layperson unfamiliar with medical and epidemiological research, their arguments can sound quite convincing. Not only do they cleverly and perversely twist scientific facts to their own advantage, but they apparently monitor every obscure meeting, journal, or media appearance to uncover statements which, taken out of context, might be used to further their cause.

One of their favorite arguments is that the evidence implicating cigarettes as a cause of disease is all statistical. Statistics, they would have us believe, are just a group of numbers looking for an argument. Yet, you would never believe that the tobacco industry businessmen did not accept statistics after looking at their annual reports, which are filled with—statistics. Why the double standard here? If statistics are acceptable to reflect financial health, why aren't they acceptable to reflect human health?

Statistics showed us the link between thalidomide taken by pregnant women and gross birth defects. Through statistics, we learned that vaccinations can protect us from polio, smallpox, and measles. Nearly everyone believes the veracity of these associations. Why should smoking be any different?

In cases where there is a long latent period between exposure to a causative agent and onset of disease, as is true for most chronic illnesses, statistics are all we have.

Of course, not every factor found in epidemiological studies to be associated with disease is necessarily a cause of that disease. Many observed associations can be spurious, occurring because of the presence of a third factor to which both the factor and the disease are related or reflecting a relationship caused by the disease itself. Epidemiologists are certainly well aware of this and make every attempt to control for such factors. On the other hand, some associations do point to cause, especially when demonstrated over and over again, and this is one of them.

Dr. Ernst Wynder, pioneer researcher in the field of tobacco and health, now Director of the American Health Foundation, once proposed a series of postulates to establish causation. Taking the relationship between smoking and lung cancer, here is how the postulates squared with the data:

1. The first postulate states that the greater and more prolonged the exposure to the factor, the greater the risk of the population involved. A substantial number of epidemiological studies have demonstrated that the greater the number of cigarettes smoked by individuals, the greater the risk of developing cancer. As you can see, there is most definitely a dose-related relationship between cigarettes smoked and lung-cancer risk.

2. The second postulate states that the epidemiological pattern should be consistent with the distribution of the factor.

The mortality rates from lung cancer in various countries correlate quite well with per capita cigarette consumption for the past three or four decades. Populations such as Mormons and Seventh-day Adventists, who do not smoke, also have very low rates of lung cancer. Most telling of all, though, is the parallel between the increase in cigarette smoking in the United States and the increase in lung cancer rates. Note that the increase in lung cancer rates among women lagged behind that of men by about thirty years—

as did their popular usage of cigarettes.

Of course, the tobacco folks love to argue that the increase in lung cancer isn't real. They insist that we may be seeing more cases of lung cancer, coincidental with the increase in cigarette smoking, simply because the methods of detecting lung cancer have improved. Techniques for detecting lung cancer have improved, but so have methods for detecting other cancers. Only for lung cancer have we seen such a dramatic increase in the past few decades.

3. Wynder's third postulate states that removal or reduction of the suspected causative factor for a given group of people should be followed by a reduction of the incidence of disease in that group. All major epidemiological studies that have examined the effects of smoking cessation have shown that people who quit smoking experience a reduction in lung-cancer risk.

Another favorite argument of the tobacco folks is that it is not smoking, but the smoker, that is the cause of the disease. They love to point out that smokers are different in many ways from nonsmokers. The industry propaganda tells us that smokers are more communicative, more energetic, more prone to drink large quantities of black coffee and liquor and to like spicy, salty food. We are also told that smokers have more marriages, more jobs, more residences, living in what you might call overdrive. They thus conclude that a smoker may also be the kind of person who is more prone to get lung cancer regardless of smoking habit. What are they trying to say? That multiple marriages, black coffee, and salt are causes of lung cancer?

Another standard industry line is that "smoking cannot

be the cause of lung cancer, heart disease, etc., because non-smokers get these diseases too." They publicize 105-year-old veteran smokers who are apparently free of smoking-related disease. This argument, is, of course, a distortion of logic and epidemiological reality. Those warning of the dangers of smoking openly acknowledge that not all smokers will develop lung cancer, heart disease, emphysema, or other cigarette-related ailments. Not everyone who runs regularly into a stream of fast moving traffic gets hit by a car. But their chances of getting hit are certainly much higher than those of a person who does not regularly dart into traffic. Obviously, there are differences in susceptibility to all types of disease—less than 2 percent of people infected with poliovirus develop paralytic polio. Not everyone exposed to the tubercule bacillus gets tuberculosis. Some people with tertiary syphillis live to a ripe old age—but most do not.

Similarly, no physician or scientist claims that tobacco use accounts for *all* causes of lung cancer, heart disease, or whatever. Drunken driving is a cause of fatal automobile accidents, but so is having your car hit by a train. The reality of multiple causation, however, should not serve to minimize or dismiss one specific cause.

Perhaps the most convincing-sounding argument used frequently by the tobacco industry is that since smoking isn't a proven cause of cancer in animals, it couldn't cause cancer in humans, either. The tobacco people are right when they say there isn't a huge amount of literature on cigarettes and animals. This is probably because animals, by some innate wisdom, do not voluntarily choose to smoke.

Yet, why would we possibly need animal studies at this stage of the game? Animal studies usually provide the *first* leads for research into human disease. For example, it was reported in 1970 that polyvinyl chloride of PVC could cause cancer in laboratory animals. *Then* epidemiological studies on high-risk human populations were launched to confirm the fact that this substance was dangerous to humans—not the other way around.

The cigarette-disease link was unique in that we began to see cancer in human populations well before there was enough suspicion to consider testing cigarettes on mice or other animals. Some animal studies have, of course, been performed and they have shown that cigarette tars cause tumors when painted on the backs of mice, and that dogs forced to smoke through a tracheal tube developed cancer-like changes in their lungs. But extensive animal testing at this time, after the fact, would seem to be redundant, given that we already know what cigarettes do to humans.

It is true that researchers are not yet sure of the exact mechanisms by which cigarette smoke causes lung cancer. Perhaps carcinogens in tobacco* act directly on target cell organs to cause changes in cells and their growth patterns. But we do not really need to know the mechanisms for causation here since the relationship is so clear.

Yes, indeed, there have been animal studies; on one of the biggest and allegedly the smartest of animals—man.

The list of arguments used by tobacco people and determined smokers goes on and on, but I think you get the picture. The "controversy" that the tobacco industry is striving so desperately to keep alive is no controversy at all.

---

*A few of the carcinogens identified in cigarette smoke: methylfluoranthrenes, benz(a)anthracene, beta-naphthylaminee, dibenzo(c)carbazole, benzo(a)pyrene, methylbenzo(a)pyrene, dimethylnitrosamine.

The Risk of Smoking

Cigarette smoking is the greatest environmental cause of death in the United States. Approximately 500,000 deaths annually are smoking-related. To put this in perspective, one out of every four deaths in this country is smoking-related. In 1992, world-renowned epidemiologist Sir Richard Doll said, "It had been thought about a quarter of smokers died from smoking-related deaths. Now we know at least a third, or maybe closer to a half of smokers die from it."

The current annual death toll from cigarette smoking worldwide is approximately 3 million, and, if present trends continue, by the year 2000 the count for this century will mount close to 100 million—a number approximately equal to the global death toll from all international warfare to date in this country.

Overall, a smoker is 70 percent more likely to die prematurely than is a comparable nonsmoker. A person who smokes two or more packs a day decreases his life expectancy by more than eight years. A one-pack-a-day smoker decreases his life expectancy by six years.

Lung cancer is the leading cause of cancer death in men and has now surpassed breast cancer as the leading cause of cancer death among women. In 1993 more than 149,000 people in the United States died of lung cancer and 90 percent of those deaths were directly attributable to smoking. Overall, male smokers are about twenty-two times more likely and female smokers over eleven times more likely to die of lung cancer than are nonsmokers.

These statistics refer to people *dying* of lung cancer rather than *getting* lung cancer for a very good reason—they are essentially the same thing. Lung cancer is one of the most incurable cancers. Seventy percent of lung cancer patients die within one year, and 87 percent are dead within five years. And it's not just old people who are victims of lung cancer. Young, beautiful cigarette smokers can be stricken in the prime of life.

It's not just lung cancer that is caused by cigarette smoking either. In fact, the Surgeon General has estimated that nearly *40 percent of all cancers* are caused by the use of tobacco products. Cigarette smoking is a major risk factor for developing cancer of the larynx, trachea, oral cavity, pharynx, esophagus, bladder, and pancreas. It is associated with increased risk of developing cancer of the cervix, kidney, and liver. There is also a synergistic effect of smoking and alcohol use that greatly increases the risk of cancer of the larynx, oral cavity, and esophagus.

Lung cancer always seems to get the most publicity as a smoking-related ailment, but it is actually not the leading cause of death in smokers. Smoking is a major risk factor for heart disease, and more people die of cigarette-related heart disease than die of cigarette-related lung cancer. Smoking nearly doubles a person's risk of heart attack. This increase in risk is less than that for lung cancer, but since heart disease is fairly common in the general population anyway, a two-fold increase in risk equals many more cases. Cigarette smoking accounts for approximately 25 percent of all heart-disease deaths.

This list of increased risks a smoker takes on is quite impressive, as is evident in the following table. It is even more impressive when you consider the fact that the smoker assumes all of these risks at the same time!

To put these risks in perspective, suppose that a doctor offered you a miracle diet pill, which would allow you to

Table 3.1
Quantifying the Risks of Smoking

HOW MANY MORE TIMES LIKELY IS A SMOKER
AT ANY PARTICULAR AGE TO DIE OF THIS DISEASE
THAN A NONSMOKER AT THE SAME AGE?

Underlying cause of death	Males	Females
Bladder cancer	3.0	2.6
Cervical cancer	—	2.1
Esophageal cancer	7.6	10.3
Kidney cancer	2.9	1.4
Laryngeal cancer	10.5	17.8
Lung cancer	22.4	11.9
Oral, lip, pharyngeal cancer	27.5	5.6
Pancreatic cancer	2.1	2.3
All causes	2.3	1.9

Note: It is important to remember that the smoker assumes all these risks at the same time. Smokers who become ill because of their cigarette smoking frequently develop more than one smoking related disease.

Source: A Report from the Surgeon General, Reducing the Health Consequences of Smoking (Rockville, Md., U.S. Department of Health and Human Services, Centers for Disease Control, Office on Smoking and Health, 1989)—DHHS Publication No. (CDC) 89-8411.

shed all those unwanted pounds effortlessly. The only catch was that the pill increased your risk of developing stomach cancer by 50 percent. Would you be interested? Probably not. A 50 percent increase in cancer risk is rather substantial, yet it pales in comparison to the risks of disease associated with smoking.

Which Substances in Cigarettes are Harmful?

More than 4,000 different substances have been identified in tobacco smoke, Scientists believe that carbon monoxide, nicotine, and "tar" are most likely to contribute to smoking's ill effects. ("Tar" is the name given to the particulate matter contained in cigarette smoke.)

There are, however, many other substances in cigarette smoke that may be harmful. These include nitrosamines, naturally occurring radioactive compounds, phenol and benzene, to name just a few. The National Cancer Institute has identified dozens of compounds in tobacco smoke known to be carcinogens or tumor promoters.

Is There Anything in Cigarettes Besides Tobacco?

Yes. In fact, much of the flavor in the low-tar and nicotine cigarettes so popular today comes from additives, rather than from tobacco. Cigarette manufacturers boast that they have more than 1,400 additives to choose from. In addition to flavorants, agents are also added to moisten the tobacco and to prevent cigarettes from self-extinguishing. These additives are not listed on cigarette packages. Nor does any government regulatory agency have any control over them, not even the Food and Drug Administration (FDA), which regulates ingredients in manufactured foods, beverages, drugs, and cosmetics.

The Comprehensive Smoking Education Act of 1984 required the tobacco industry to provide the Department of Health and Human Services with a partial list of additives used in cigarettes, conduct research on the additives' safety, and report the findings back to Congress. However, this information is of dubious value, as the list remains confidential. There are little data to indicate whether many of these additives are safe when burned. No government entity has the authority to restrict or eliminate any of the additives.

Available data suggest that at last some of these additives are not safe when burned. Cocoa, for example, is a common cigarette additive which is harmless when eaten. However, animal tests indicate that it may be carcinogenic when burned. Certain sugars, which are often used to flavor cigarettes, produce a substance called catechol when heateed. Catechol is a major co-carcinogen in tobacco smoke. Licorice extract is added to tobacco to improve flavor and keep tobacco moist. Glycyrrhizic acid, the active component of licorice, is a precursor to carcinogenic polycyclic hydrocarbons when burned. Glycerols and glycols, which are tobacco additives used to keep tobacco moist, produce a compound called acrolein when burned. Acrolein is extremely irritating and has been shown to interfere with the normal clearing of the lungs. Recent research shows that acrolein acts like a carcinogen, though not yet classified as such, and produces changes in the cells of human bronchial mucosa. In addition, menthol, one of the most common ingredients in cigarettes, is an anesthetic, acting to numb the throats of smokers, which is the real reason smokers find mentholated cigarettes to be "cooler."

Judging from the limited amount of information we have about cigarette additives, it appears that there is ample cause for concern over their unrestricted use.

Smokeless Tobacco

While snuff dipping and tobacco chewing have traditionally been relegated to the backwoods, the lone prairie, and the outfield, over the past two decades the smokeless tobacco habit has moved into mainstream America. (See box below). Colleges from coast to coast now sport tobacco chewing clubs and the circular imprint of a snuff tin on the rear blue jean pocket has become de rigeur for many junior high and high school students across the country. Smokeless tobacco product use has almost tripled from 1972 through 1991.

Chew and Snuff

There are four types of chewing tobacco: loose leaf, fine cut, plug, and twist.

The most popular of the chewing products is loose leaf, which is made almost entirely from cigar-leaf tobacco. It is sold in small packages and may be heavily flavored or plain. Fine cut is similar but is more finely cut, so that it resembles snuff. Plug is leaf tobacco that has been pressed into flat cakes and sweetened by molasses, licorice, maple sugar, honey, or the like. Twist is made from stemmed leaves twisted into small rolls and folded. These tobacco "chews" are not really chewed, but held between the cheek and lower jaw.

Snuff may be dry or moist and is often sweetened, flavored, salted, and/or scented. At one time, snuff was sniffed (or snuffed) through the nose, hence its name. Now it is generally "dipped" by tucking a pinch between the gum and lower lip. (One company has begun marketing snuff in handy tea-baglike pouches, advising consumers to "take a pouch instead of a puff.")

The tobacco and its juices must, of course, be disposed of periodically. (Swallowing the tobacco or its juices can have dire consequences. As one writer observes, swallow a little and you don't want to eat; swallow a lot and you don't want to live.) In some areas, the disposal of tobacco juices has become quite stylized. On one college campus, for example, it is considered "in" to spit into a Campbell's soup can.

In 1991, an estimated 5.3 million U.S. adults were current users of smokeless tobacco and 7.9 million former users. Worse yet, a Centers for Disease Control and Prevention (CDC) survey of twenty-two states revealed that nearly one in five males in grades nine to twelve are currently using smokeless or spit tobacco. Many users start at an alarmingly young age—one-third of those interviewed by CDC began as early as five years of age, with the average age of first use being just nine.

Spit tobacco use is astronomically high among athletes. its use increased dramatically—by 40 percent—among college athletes between 1985 and 1989. Use in baseball has gone up from 45 percent to 57 percent; football, up from 30 percent to 40 percent; and even in tennis from 12 percent to 29 percent. Most college athletes began the habit well before their college days.

Even though television advertising of smokeless tobacco was banned with the passage of the Comprehensive Smokeless Tobacco Health Education Act of 1986, the use of smokeless tobacco products continues to rise. At least 50 million pounds of moist snuff alone—just one form of smokeless tobacco—was used in 1992.

Why is it that smokeless tobacco use has gained such popularity and acceptance? One of the most compelling reasons is that it has become socially acceptable in communities across the country, not just in rural areas but in elite urban areas as well. Former surgeon general Antonia Novello, M.D., said in 1992 that parents mistakenly think it is much safer than smoking; school officials agree that at least it isn't cigarettes. And kids view it as the ultimate "cool" activity.

Another powerful influence is baseball: by 1991, at least

45 percent of professional baseball players chewed. In June of 1993, smokeless tobacco use was banned in the minor league, with the philosophy that baseball players greatly influence kids. What's the scoop here? Why ban it in the minors when kids watch and idolize the major league players?

Smokeless tobacco companies continue exceptionally clever marketing schemes. Not only do they frequently place smokeless tobacco products in close proximity to candies and snacks, but they influence the availability of candy products that are "chew look-alikes." A shredded bubble gum called "Big League Chew" and sunflower seeds marketed as "Dugout Chew" are big sellers, and often gateway products into the real thing.

According to 1990 reports by the Federal Trade Commission, spit tobacco companies spent $35 million of their $104 million advertising budgets—over one-third—on public entertainment and distributing free samples. The activities and images portrayed in these promotions are designed to appeal to young males, especially those under the age of eighteen. Chew manufacturers sponsor auto races, rodeos, monster truck shows, tractor pulls, and country music concerts. All activities they sponsor are associated with the outdoors or sports, often with entertainment stars and touting independence and rebellion.

Many people who chew tobacco believe they are spared the dangers of tobacco because they aren't smoking it. Nothing could be further from the truth. The cancer risk of using smokeless tobacco looms just as large as it does for smoking. Furthermore, CDC research released in 1993 revealed that one-fourth of smokeless tobacco users also smoke, placing themselves in double jeopardy. Indeed, cigarette smoking actually increased slightly among adolescent boys from the early 1980s to the early 1990s, the very group most likely to use spit tobacco.

Those who use smokeless tobacco are at extremely high risk for gum and cheek lesions or sores that lead to cancer. About 75 percent of oral and throat cancers are attributed to the use of such tobacco. Frighteningly, there is just a 50 percent five-year survival rate for such cancers. In addition, many who do survive such cancers have an exceptionally high risk of developing subsequent cancers.

In addition to the cancer risk, there are other health perils. Contrary to popular belief, smokeless tobacco is addicting— and rapidly so. The amount of nicotine a snuff user absorbs by consuming eight to ten dips per day is equivalent to that consumed by heavy cigarette smokers. In the CDC's 1992 survey, young people used spit tobacco an average of six times per day, and more than one-fourth used it ten times or more each day—the nicotine equivalent of one to two packs of cigarettes. And because users keep the wad or pinch in the mouth for twenty to thirty minutes at a time, the average spit-tobacco user absorbs a greater amount of nicotine than does the average cigarette smoker.

Heart disease is another risk associated with smokeless tobacco use. Pregnant women who use it expose their unborn babies to the same nicotine as does a cigarette smoker. According to the CDC's 1993 report, other suggested health problems include upper-digestive-tract cancers, high blood pressure, and cancers of the throat, pancreas, prostate in males, and urinary tract.

It should be obvious that smokeless tobacco use is not the harmless, fun habit that many people would like to believe it is.

Is Second-Hand Smoke *Really* a Threat to Our Health?

Earlier this year, the Environmental Protection Agency released its long-awaited report assessing the health risks of other people's cigarette smoke—"Environmental Tobacco Smoke (ETS)." Their conclusion: ETS causes 3,000 cases of lung cancer annually in nonsmokers; is responsible for hundreds of thousands of cases of bronchitis and pneumonia in children; and induces or worsens asthma in up to one million young Americans. (ETS contributions to heart disease were not considered in this report, but may be addressed later.) The public health community welcomed the official findings, noting they were consistent with other scientific reviews.

The tobacco industry—which has, for over forty years, been blowing smoke by officially dismissing the causal link between active smoking and premature disease and death—responded with denials and accusations that the EPA study was the product of a fanatical antismoking movement that was manipulating data to advance their ultimate agenda—universal restrictions on smoking. Recently, the industry filed suit against the EPA in federal court in Greensboro, North Carolina, requesting that the judge declare the classification of ETS as a "Class A" carcinogen "null and void."

Is there scientific evidence that passive or second-hand smoke is a health hazard? Or is the EPA conclusion yet another example of government-inspired "science fiction" engineered, in this case, by those who are waging an ideological vendetta against the tobacco industry?

SCIENTIFIC CREDIBILITY

The EPA has a dismal record in separating real health risks from bogus ones. It was this agency that slapped the designation "probable human carcinogen" on the apple growth regulator Alar four years ago and contributed to the great Apple Panic of 1989. The Alar apple scare was later shown to be scientifically baseless. The EPA oversees the Superfund program which targets "cancer causing" dumpsites. Yet, there is no evidence that such sites pose any cancer risk at all. It was the EPA that called for the evacuation of Times Beach, Missouri, at a cost of about $20 million, touting the hypothetical risk of dioxin.

So when EPA calls ETS a "Class A carcinogen" (meaning there is human evidence that it causes cancer), skeptics from both the business and scientific communities (myself included) wondered whether this was not just more environmental hype. But, just as past crimes cannot be admitted as evidence in a current trial, we cannot judge the EPA because it has overstated or misrepresented risks in the past. We must judge them on the current facts.

PLAUSIBILITY

Theoretically, one could advance the opinion that anything—say fax machines or Kleenex—causes cancer. But to be taken seriously, such claims need a biological hypothesis, a scientific context in which they make sense. Clearly the hypothesis that ETS causes human cancer *does* have that biological context. Second-hand smoke has essentially the same chemical components as direct smoke, and we know beyond any reasonable doubt that direct smoke dramatically increases the risk of cancer of the lung, bladder, pancreas, cervix, esophagus, and other sites. Active smoking increases cancer risk even at low doses of exposure, five to ten cigarettes per day, a level of carcinogen exposure that may be in the same range as high dose ETS exposure. (At least one published autopsy study confirmed that nonsmokers married to smokers frequently have precancerous lesions on their lungs.) But is there evidence that ETS is present at sufficiently high doses to cause cancer? (The arguments that passive inhalation is less hazardous than primary smoking because smoke gets filtered through the nose rather than being taken directly into the lungs from the mouth have now been dismissed because researchers have found that ETS particles are so small that they escape the nasal filtering system and also enter the lungs directly.)

EXPOSURE

In evaluating this question, scientists have examined heavily exposed nonsmokers, specifically the most readily available data base—nonsmoking women married to smokers. Despite the denials of the tobacco industry and a few independent commentators, the overwhelming number of published "spouse studies" indicate that these high-risk women have an increased risk of lung cancer. Admittedly, it is a relatively small increased risk compared to direct smoking. Twenty-four of thirty studies evaluated by EPA found an increased risk, although not all were statistically significant. (The much-publicized criticism of the EPA panel using a 90 percent confidence level as opposed to a 95 percent one is a statistical red herring. Any qualified statistician looking at the published data will agree that the findings of a slightly increased lung cancer risk in nonsmoking women did not occur by chance.) The industry argues, in desperation, that a late 1992 study was omitted, thus biasing the EPA conclusion. Actually, the study in question was published after the cut-off period and, ironically, would have provided only more support for the EPA findings. The authors noted: "Ours and other recent studies suggest a small but consistent increased risk of lung cancer from passive smoking."

Perhaps the most neutral evaluation of the cancer risk of passive smoking comes from Sir Richard Doll of the University of Oxford, who is not specifically known as an antismoking activist and is highly regarded by many epidemiologists as the current "dean" of our medical discipline. When I asked him for his assessment on ETS, he wrote, "The [World Health Organization] agreed some six or seven years before the EPA that environmental tobacco smoke must be accepted as a human carcinogen. There is a real problem estimating the quantitative effect of environmental tobacco smoke. [But] the suggestion that environmental tobacco smoke is not a human carcinogen can be dismissed as devoid of scientific basis."

As to the noncancer risks, including asthma and other respiratory distress, incurred by nonsmokers, particularly children, the evidence is overwhelming and unequivocal. Children of smokers have higher rates of illness and more school absenteeism. The vast majority of childhood middle-ear infections are caused by parental smoking. Staggering health care costs result from the hospitalizations and surgeries (the most common pediatric type) that these infections necessitate. Interestingly, the tobacco industry has not even attempted to deny these data. Philip Morris spokesman Steve Parish agrees that people "should not blow smoke in the face of children. People should use some common sense."

WHAT SHOULD WE DO?

In a January 1993 speech, Michael A. Miles, Chairman of Philip Morris (maker of Marlboros and other tobacco products), likened the ETS "scare" to the unfounded panics about the cancer-inducing effects of Alar, dioxin, and chlorine. Similarly, John Berry, legal counsel for the Council for Burley Tobacco, a party to the lawsuit against EPA, charged, "The EPA destroyed the town of Times Beach, Missouri, with exaggerated scare tactics on dioxin. If the court does not act in our favor, communities throughout Kentucky . . . will also be destroyed by a government agency that has, quite simply, run amok."

But their analogies comparing trace levels of environmental chemical exposures with ETS fail. The risks of Alar and chlorine in food and water, and dioxin in soil, are purely hypothetical with data derived from limited animal studies. The cancer risks of ETS, however small, are real. The data are based on human observations.

Clearly, the health risks of ETS are dose-related. People who live daily in an environment of cigarette smoke are the ones most at risk. Ironically, then, the most risk exists where regulators have no control—in the home. (Increasingly, judges in divorce settlements are taking parental smoking habits into account when assigning custody.) But other areas of high-dose exposure could be the workplace, schools, day-care centers, air and ground conveyances, and basically anywhere people may be exposed daily over many years. But how much ETS is too much to tolerate, and who decides? This—not the question of whether ETS causes human cancer—is the true area of controversy and debate.

The lifetime risk that a nonsmoking woman married to

a smoker will develop lung cancer from ETS is estimated to be 1 in 500, as compared to a chance of about 1 in 10 of developing lung cancer from active smoking. But given that the risks of active smoking are so astronomically high compared to other life risks, it is inappropriate to compare passive smoking with the active form. It is better to compare ETS risk with other known human environmental cancer risks, for example, asbestos.

It is possible to argue that we should not tolerate any level of a carcinogen and that to avoid cancer risk, smoking should be banned in all public places. On the other hand, it is the dose that makes the poison, and transient exposures (such as in a fast food restaurant) might thus be irrelevant to lung cancer causation, but not necessarily irrelevant to the causation and exacerbation of acute respiratory distress. Exposures to ETS, however, are cumulative and omnipresent for many of us. The levels of ETS in our lives today far exceed legally tolerated levels of other known human carcinogens—like asbestos—in our highly regulated society.

The question no longer is whether ETS causes lung cancer—it does. The question for the society that takes a regulatory exorcist approach to trace levels of *hypothetical carcinogens* is: At what level will we tolerate a *known human carcinogen?*

Who Are Today's Smokers?

Although the rate of smoking has declined significantly since the mid-1960s, there are still some 50 million smokers in the United States—about the same number as twenty years ago. Currently, about 32 percent of American men and 27 percent of American women smoke cigarettes. These figures represent a significant drop in the rate of smoking among men, from a maximum rate of over 50 percent. The smoking rate for women has declined by only a few percentage points over the years, however, from a peak of 33 percent in 1965.

Smoking is inversely related to income and occupational level. Individuals in white-collar positions are less likely to smoke than are blue-collar workers. The difference in smoking rates is greater for men than for women. In addition, evidence indicates that male blue-collar workers are less likely to quit successfully than their white-collar counterparts.

Educational level seems to be another important factor related to smoking behavior. In general, the more highly educated a person is, the less likely he or she is to smoke, although, again, the relationship is stronger for men than for women. Smoking prevalence among college graduates has decreased from 34 percent in 1966 to 16 percent in 1987. In contrast, the smoking level among high school graduates decreased from 41 percent in 1966 to 33 percent in 1987, less than half the reduction shown by college graduates. Individuals without high school diplomas show no appreciable decline in smoking levels.

Are some teenagers more likely to smoke than others? It appears so. A study of high school seniors conducted by the National Institute on Drug Abuse (NIDA) indicated that students who did not perform well academically were more likely to smoke than were academically successful students. Students who smoked were also more likely to be enrolled in vocational courses, rather than in a college-preparatory curriculum. Overall, the educational and occupational aspirations of high school students who smoked tended to be lower than those of nonsmoking students. Teenagers who live in single-parent homes or whose parents, siblings, or friends smoke were found to be more apt to take up smoking. However, focusing solely on the behaviors and attributes of teenagers who smoke neglects an important component of the problem—cigarette advertising.

Pushing Tobacco on Our Children

Tobacco companies specifically target advertising to children. They need to attract young people, and get them addicted at an early age, to replace the half a million customers who die each year as a direct result of smoking cigarettes and the more than one million who quit. A case in point is the shameless use of cartoon characters to promote smoking as "cool" and essential to popularity. Teenage girls are subject to the added and possibly more insidious message that "smoking keeps you slim" by advertisements depicting young, beautiful, thin, and fashionably dressed models celebrating their "liberation" by smoking cigarettes.

A new twist in luring young girls to smoke came from the makers of Virginia Slims in March 1993. They advertised a new feminine "fashion collection with a streetwise attitude." The clothes embody the look that any young, carefree, fun-loving woman would just die for: a black biker jacket with coordinated vest, bracelet, V-neck tie, belt bag, backpack, and sunglasses. The clothes were advertised as "free" with the purchase of just under 980 packages of Virginia Slims; one had to submit proofs of purchase by the manufacturer, Philip Morris, by August 31, 1993. That averaged just over five packs of cigarettes per day for the six months of the promotion. To average five packs per day one would have to smoke one cigarette every eight minutes during waking hours. The fact that Philip Morris gets away with this type of outrageously deceptive advertising is just another example of the privileged status the industry enjoys.

It should be no surprise, then, that more than 90 percent of all cigarette smokers began smoking before age twenty, with more than 2 million Americans becoming addicted to nicotine each year. The average age for the very first use of cigarettes is thirteen years. Over 3,000 teenagers become regular smokers each day in the United States. Teenage girls, in particular, are starting to smoke at an early age—young women under the age of twenty-three are the only age group showing a rise in smoking rates. A recent study estimated that the tobacco industry enjoys a profit of approximately $221 million from sales of cigarettes to children under the age of eighteen.

About one billion packs of cigarettes are sold annually to minors through retailers and vending machines. No other type of drug pushing to teenagers is more blatant, widespread, or profitable. But most national and state government officials have chosen to ignore the outrageous activities of tobacco pushers, which will probably result in 100 times more deaths than those caused by cocaine and heroin combined. Finally, studies indicate that smoking acts as a "gateway drug," because it is associated with increased use of alcohol and illicit drugs among teenagers.

Is Cigarette Smoking Addictive?

The 1988 Surgeon General's Report concluded that cigarettes and other forms of tobacco are addicting. Nicotine is the drug in tobacco responsible for that addiction. The report also concluded that the processes which determine heroin and cocaine addiction are similar to those of nicotine addiction. This physical addiction is bolstered by the behavioral and psychological components involved in the cigarette habit.

Surveys indicate that 90 percent of smokers would like to quit. Eighty to 85 percent of those who have tried, however, say that they have relapsed within three months. These figures indicate that *the majority of smokers smoke, not because they want to, but because they are unable to give it up.*

Research implicates nicotine as an important factor in establishing and maintaining tobacco dependency, although there is also a strong behavioral or psychological component involved.

When cigarette smoke is inhaled, about 25 percent of its nicotine reaches the brain within six seconds. The average smoker who smokes a pack and a half a day consumes 10,950 cigarettes per year. At an average of ten puffs per cigarette, the smoker gets 109,000 nicotine surges per year. No other form of drug use occurs with such frequency and regularity.

During cigarette smoking the heart rate and blood pressure increase. Initially the smoker feels more alert and performs better on memory and learning tasks, but it is not clear if this is an effect that brings the smoker above baseline or if it merely restores equilibrium to the smoker in a mild state of nicotine withdrawal.

Smokers generally experience withdrawal when they quit. Physiological changes that accompany smoking cessation include decreased heart rate, increased blood pressure, and brain-wave changes. Those who quit smoking often initially demonstrate impaired performance on coordination tests and decreased ability to concentrate. Sleep disturbances, irritability, anxiety, and gastrointestinal disturbances also may occur.

Most important, many individuals who give up smoking experience severe, often overpowering cravings for tobacco.

RECENT DEVELOPMENTS

As we go to press, facts about the addictive nature of nicotine are appearing in the news. On February 28, 1994, "Day One," a magazine show produced by ABC News, aired an exposé on the tobacco industry's manipulation of nicotine. The "Day One" story and the FDA's own findings illustrate for the first time publicly exactly what the tobacco industry is capable of—the manipulation of the amount and even the presence of nicotine in cigarettes. The potential implication of the new disclosures is substantial for many reasons including:

- *The FDA's rationale for not regulating the contents, manufacture, sale, or advertising of tobacco products has been based largely on the concept that they are neither foods nor drugs.* If the FDA concludes that nicotine is not an inevitable component of tobacco products and that it is being consciously manipulated to affect the impact of tobacco products on consumers, the agency may regulate nicotine-containing tobacco products as drugs pursuant to the Food, Drug, and Cosmetic Act. The FDA already exercises its authority to regulate the use of nicotine, the advertising of products containing nicotine, and the sale of products containing nicotine for all products containing nicotine, *except* tobacco products. The FDA is now seeking "guidance" from Congress on how to proceed.

- *The revelation that tobacco manufacturers and suppliers to the manufacturers manipulate nicotine could influence the public's perception of these products and the companies that make them.* It is one thing to manufacture a harmful product which happens to contain an addictive substance, but it is quite another to deliberately manipulate the addictive substance with the intent to hook consumers.

- *Tobacco manufacturers have the capability to remove all or virtually all of the nicotine from their tobacco products* using technology which is already in place and in use. Nicotine need no longer be a "necessary" component of a cigarette product.

Health advocates' predictions that the nicotine manipulation story may result in dramatic changes in the tobacco and health policy environment have been echoed by the tobacco industry itself. Philip Morris recently brought a $10 billion libel suit against ABC in response to airing of the nicotine manipulation story. The industry feels that the showing of tobacco manufacturers' deliberate manipulation of nicotine does indeed appear to have the potential to dramatically change the product liability scene as it affects smoker death lawsuits.

Alternative Ways to Use Tobacco are Also Dangerous

Some smokers, rightfully concerned about the health hazards of smoking, believe they can reduce their risk of tobacco-related disease by switching to "safer," alternative methods of tobacco use instead of quitting. However, no form of tobacco use is without risk—tobacco is tobacco is tobacco. The best way to avoid tobacco-associated disease is to avoid using tobacco in any form.

Low-tar, low-nicotine cigarettes. There is no evidence demonstrating any significant reduction in risk for smoking-induced disease by switching to low tar, low nicotine brands. In fact studies indicate that many smokers unconsciously increase the number of cigarettes they smoke, inhale more deeply or take more puffs on each cigarette when they switch to a low tar, low nicotine brand in order to keep their nicotine intake constant.

Pipe and cigar smoking. There are definite health risks associated with smoking cigars and pipes, although not as dramatic and extensive as those associated with cigarette smoking. Generally, cigar and pipe smokers smoke less than cigarette smokers and inhale less deeply. But even many of those who inhale minimally suffer tobacco-induced disease.

The harmful effects of pipe and cigar smoking are concentrated at those body sites directly exposed to the smoke. Pipe and cigar smokers have as high a risk as cigarette smokers of dying of cancer of the mouth, larynx, throat, and esophagus. Pipe and cigar smokers have somewhat higher death rates from some other smoking-related diseases than do nonsmokers, but lower rates than cigarette smokers.

There is, however, no evidence that either pipe or cigar smoke per se is any less dangerous than cigarette smoke. Among populations who inhale cigar smoke, available scientific evidence suggests that the overall health risks are similar to those incurred by cigarette smokers, and people who switch from cigarettes to pipes or cigars are especially likely to inhale the smoke from the latter.

I've Been Smoking for Twenty Years. Is It Still Worthwhile for Me to Quit or Has the Damage Been Done?

No matter how long you've smoked, how old you are, or your current state of health, it is still beneficial to quit. The 1990 Surgeon General's Report cited "major and immediate" health benefits of smoking cessation for men and women of every age group. For example, ex-smokers reduce their risk of smoking-related coronary heart disease by 50 percent within one year of quitting. After fifteen years of abstinence, their risk is similar to that of lifetime nonsmokers. Former smokers live longer than continuing smokers and enjoy reduced risk of lung cancer, other cancers, heart disease, stroke, and chronic lung disease.

The health benefits of smoking cessation are not limited by age or health status. The benefits of quitting extend to persons older than sixty years. An otherwise healthy man aged sixty to sixty-four who quits smoking reduces his risk of dying in the next fifteen years by ten percent. Persons with smoking-related disease can experience important health benefits through quitting. These include reduced risk of recurrent heart attack and related death for those with diagnosed coronary heart disease and reduced risk of respiratory infections such as pneumonia, which are frequently the immediate causes of death in patients with chronic disease.

Why Do People Keep Smoking?

A MALEVOLENT WEB

How can a product as dangerous as the cigarette continue to be accepted—and indeed be heavily promoted by advertising—in such a health-conscious and demanding society? Why are there not frequent television documentaries, investigative reports, outraged citizens groups, and concerned legislatures dealing with what is unarguably the most dramatic and far-reaching public health threat of this century? Why do we have anxious scrutiny over traces of dioxin, yet apathy about cigarettes as a cause of disease? How, thirty years after the cigarette was definitely shown to be a health hazard, does the tobacco industry remain triumphant in its knowledge of a secure future? The answer lies in a malevolent web of five extrinsic and intrinsic factors:

- The happenstance of a cruel and unpredictable backfire in human innovation.

- The physically addictive nature of cigarettes, which keeps smokers hooked despite a desire to quit.

- The human tendency to reject the premise that, under some circumstances, we may be responsible for causing our own illness or death—the adaptive psychological defense mechanisms allowing the smoker to sublimate, repress, and disassociate him- or herself from the bad news about cigarettes.

- The related reluctance of nonsmokers to bring up grim statistics when they know that the smoker is already overburdened with guilt and anxiety.

- The enormous and unprecedented economic clout and lobbying effort exerted by the tobacco industry. Those dependent on it for their livelihood take great pains to ensure that their addicted and potentially addicted customers are shielded from frequent onslaughts of information about how harmful cigarette smoking is.

BACKFIRE

It goes without saying that, if the cigarette were being considered for introduction today, there is no way it would meet the safety criteria of either the Food and Drug Administration or the Consumer Product Safety Commission, the two agencies most logical for approving and regulating it. Even without the dozens of human studies we have today, these agencies would reject cigarettes because burned tobacco contains a significant number of cancer-causing agents and the immediate effects of tobacco inhalation (increased heart rate, increase in blood carbon monoxide levels, inhibition of stomach contractions) would be sufficient causes of concern. Whether it was the small businessman trying to have cigarettes approved or a large corporation's research department that came up with this "brainstorm," today the cigarette would not make its way out of the federal testing laboratories, and the economic impact of the nonapproval of cigarettes would be negligible.

However, the cigarette is not just being introduced; it has been around for approximately one hundred years. (Tobacco, of course, has been used for generations, but it was the invention of the cigarette manufacturing machine in the 1880s that resulted in a new and devastating form of behavior—inhalation of smoke on a regular basis, directly into the lungs.)

Through the first sixty years of its hundred-year existence, the cigarette and the marking techniques that went with it represented a stellar success for those who worked hard and ingeniously in a free enterprise environment to sell a product that purportedly gave pleasure, prestige, and relaxation to millions of eager customers. During the first six decades, there was, of course, "controversy" about cigarettes, and eventually some impressive scientific evidence indicating that cigarettes were hazardous. In general, however, the period between 1890 and 1950 marked the golden age of the cigarette, the birth of a new symbol of the all-American man and woman. That was the dream: the carefree life; the glamorous ads; the hints that cigarettes might not only be pleasurable, but even healthful; and the development of a major, successful economic base for millions of people, directly or indirectly financially dependent on the production, manufacture, sales, and advertising of cigarettes.

Then, in 1950, the dream became a nightmare. In a near explosion of medical data, smokers and nonsmokers alike were jolted by the reports of the devastating health impact of the pleasure-giving cigarette. The news was, quite decidedly, too frightening to fully digest, and indeed, through much of the 1950s, the most prevalent reaction of the medical profession, the press, and the general public was to downplay the evidence, demand "further data," point to alleged gaps and limitations of the "statistics," and run as far from the reality as possible. Human innovation had backfired, and people did not know what to do about it. For years, honest, hard-working, enterprising Americans had grown tobacco, manufactured cigarettes, and promoted and distributed the product in a clever (and well-intentioned) manner. The tragedy here is that, by the time the bad news about cigarettes had accumulated, the cigarette had become socially desirable and enormous segments of the economic system—including the U.S. government—were dependent on the cigarette as a source of revenue. Not least of all, a sizable portion of the American population was already physically addicted to the product.

ADDICTION

Most Americans are well aware of the addictive properties of illegal "recreational" drugs like heroin. Many would be shocked to learn that Dr. William Polin, Director of the National Institute on Drug Abuse, terms cigarette smoking "the most widespread drug dependence in our country. " As we mentioned earlier, given that the average smoker consumes 10,950 cigarettes per year and puffs each ten times, that smoker gets 109,000 doses of nicotine per year. There is no other form of drug abuse that comes close to this frequency and regularity.

The evidence on the addictive nature of smoking is evident in national surveys indicating that 90 percent of smokers would like to quit and that 85 percent have tried to quit, but failed. Cigarette smokers are physiological prisoners, their bodies in need of the substances in cigarette smoke in order to perform efficiently. Repeated studies indicate that tobacco is more addictive than heroin, producing very strong physical dependence. Cigarette withdrawal symptoms include significant body changes leading to decrease in heart rate, increase in appetite, disturbances in sleep patterns, anxiety, irritability, and aggressiveness.

When smokers tell you that they have tried to stop smoking, but just can't, they really mean it. Moreover, of those who *are* able to give up smoking, some 70 percent resume the habit within three months—about the same recidivism rate as heroin. One cannot overstate the contribution that this addictive nature has made to the continued use of the cigarette; indeed, it is an essential component of the tobacco industry's recipe for survival.

PSYCHOLOGICAL BLACKOUT

The survival of the cigarette into the 1990s is testimony to the existence of the psychological mechanisms that protect us from facts with which we cannot cope. The classic response to cognitive dissonance, which occurs when people acquire new information that clashes with their current behavior or firmly held belief, was vividly evident during the 1950s. That's when retrospective human epidemiological studies around the world confirmed the extraordinary rates of lung cancer, heart disease, emphysema, and other ailments among smokers. People simply refused to incorporate this new information into their consciousness. During that entire decade, there was enormous resistance on the part of the media, legislators, and even physicians to believe the new findings, and a tendency to dismiss what was unacceptable.

Today's surveys show that 90 percent of Americans know cigarette smoke is hazardous to health (although most of them "know" it only in the rhetorical sense, unaware of the specific dangers). The clash here is between the reality of smoking and the evidence available that it is harmful. The two beliefs cannot exist together, so it is the evidence that is repressed and in some cases sublimated. (For example, some smokers declare their "health consciousness" by joining an exercise club or shopping at a "health food" store, but continue to smoke.)

In plain English, smokers do not want to talk or think about the dangers of their habit. Currently, public service advertisements about the hazards of smoking are few and far between, so most smokers find it relatively easy to avoid mental dissonance. Cigarette smoking literally becomes an involuntary, automatic form of behavior, with no incentive for the smoker to reevaluate his or her decision to smoke from week to week.

Researchers are currently investigating another psychological explanation for cigarette addiction. Recent studies indicate that depression may be a missing link in understanding the chain of dependence. The personality of the smoker, for example, may predispose him or her to depression. A genetic link may also exist between smoking behavior and depression. In addition, smokers may use nicotine as an aid to altering their mood states. In individuals prone to depression, such a neutral emotional state is highly desired and, perhaps, only achieved through the use of drugs. Smokers predisposed to depression are also less successful in their cessation efforts.

NONSMOKERS' RELUCTANCE

It would seem logical that the nonsmoker, unencumbered by the physiological addiction to cigarettes, would be an ideal source of encouragement for smoking cessation. However, it generally does not work that way, because some basic human psychological mechanisms are at work.

First, disease data on smoking are so horrifying that it may be difficult for a wife, for example, to allow herself to even imagine her husband experiencing an excruciating death from lung cancer, and a type of "secondhand" denial may set in. Second, she might meet major resistance and strike a chord of marital dissension should she attempt to focus her smoking husband on the subject. Third, in dealing with a friend, relative, or anyone else who smokes, many nonsmokers sense the smoker's depression, guilt, and unhappiness, sometimes masked by one-liners and grim humor, and feel reluctant to make a bad situation worse by bringing up such a depressing topic. There are, inevitably, many relatives, friends, and employers seriously concerned about the health of their smoking friends, but simply baffled about how to tactfully, graciously, and effectively bring the topic up without incurring the wrath of the person they are trying to help.

The combination of the "guilt-ridden smoker's phenomenon" and the helplessness of the nonsmoker in giving the advice may be one reason why certain institutions—like churches and synagogues—have generally ignored the topic. This is ironic since, while religious organizations across the country may differ widely in their codes of theology, all are united in their belief that human life is precious. Most probably would agree that it is a sin, however defined, to take one's own life. Many have taken formal stances on potentially life-threatening aspects of lifestyle. For example, the National Council of Churches of Christ has issued official policy statements on drug abuse, health care, and alcohol use, but it and almost all other formal religious sects in this country maintain silence on the subject of cigarettes and health. (A vivid exception here is the Seventh-Day Adventists Church, which issues a substantial quantity of literature about the dangers of smoking, complete with photographs of diseased lungs.)

Why would a clergyman who grimly warned you that shooting yourself in the head with a loaded pistol would be contrary to God's wishes not warn you that slow-motion suicide was equally unacceptable and immoral? Why would the National Council of Churches take on the issue of infant formula in the Third World claiming that it was life-threatening, and then turn their heads on a practice that kills hundreds of thousands of Americans, and is about to kill millions of new smokers in developing nations? The answer again indicates the physiological addiction process. It also points to the fact that a sizable minority of clergymen, like everyone else, smokes cigarettes. Finally, many perceive the smoking problem to be so deep-rooted and hopeless that no effort is made to address the subject.

Part of the psychological cover-up on the subject of smoking might be explained by the human eagerness to blame misfortune on anyone but ourselves. In the case of Third World feeding practices, the "enemy" was the infant formula manufacturers; in the case of the anxiety about the health effects of dioxin or Red Dye #2, the "villain" is the chemical. It is far easier to focus one's attention and ire on health risks imposed by outside forces than it is to become introspective about one's own role in human disease. This rejection of introspection may, for example, explain the total lack of interest in the subject of cigarettes among the "women's movement" as represented by the National Organization for Women (NOW) and other groups with a commitment to improving the quality of women's lives. The movement has been both active and successful in reducing on-the-job discrimination, fostering equal opportunity in advanced education, reducing the gap in compensation between males and females, proclaiming women's rights to control their own bodies by encouraging birth control and abortion availability, and developing novel ways of effectively combining careers with family life. It thus seems a bit strange that there is a peculiar silence on the subject of women's smoking in feminist circles.

The feminist health "bible," *Our Bodies, Ourselves,* has only a passing reference to the subject of smoking. When asked about this, Judy Norsigian, a member of the Boston Women's Health Collective that produced the original book, explained they had intended to include a chapter on smoking, alcohol, and drugs, but "there was not sufficient room in the book, and we did not have the resources to do the research." The National Women's Health Network, which represents about 1,000 American women's health organizations, has "no formal position on smoking." The San Francisco Women's Health Collective, an organization describing itself as devoted to "women's health education," does not address the smoking issue because "it [is] not a priority in terms of health education."

Even the magazines of "liberated" women stand mute on this subject. The former *Ms.* magazine, which claimed to "serve women as people, not roles," had distinct opinions about what advertising it should accept and was on record as saying it would not accept advertising that is offensive to women (for example, they turned down ads for vaginal deodorants), but would freely advertise cigarettes and never carried an article on smoking and health.

Why the silence here? In the case of the magazines, it is clear that the advertising revenue from tobacco companies plays some role, but there must be more to it than that. Feminist groups have a tradition of focusing on problems they feel are unique to women, and perhaps they unconsciously decided that the cigarette problem affected everyone. However, in the 1990s with lung cancer replacing breast cancer as the leading cause of cancer death in women and cigarettes being the major controllable threat to the health of unborn children, should not priorities be reexamined? That is where the addiction and "self-inflicted" nature of the cigarette nightmare comes in. Once again, the major thrust of the women's movement has always been focused on what others (particularly the male of the species) are doing to women, as opposed to what they are doing to themselves. In order to effectively address the growing calamity of cigarettes in women's death and morbidity, the leaders of the feminist movement must for once become introspective, acknowledging that the cigarette problem is largely self-induced.

ECONOMIC CLOUT AND LOBBYING EFFORTS

Tobacco, particularly in the form of cigarettes, *is* Big Business in the United States. Not only is tobacco grown in twenty-two American states and our sixth largest cash crop, but there is a vast and complex tobacco supply network that extends the chain of economic dependence on tobacco to include a full spectrum of industries, including manufacturers of farm supplies and equipment, transportation, advertising, and, in turn, those who depend on these suppliers. Thus, the economic ripple effect extends from the tobacco manufacturers, to Madison Avenue ad agencies, and finally to newspapers and magazines that derive billions of dollars annually in revenues from cigarette ads. In addition, any list of "cigarette dependents" must include federal, state, and local governments, which yearly receive billions of dollars in cigarette sales and excise taxes.

There are four major ways that tobacco interests flex their economic muscle when they perceive any threat to their most important product—cigarettes. First, they rely on the corporate clout of their family companies. By buying soft drink, insurance, food, and alcoholic beverage companies, they have succeeded in spreading even further the economic dependency on cigarettes, thus extending the reach of their corporate teeth. For example, Del Monte, which operates canneries and specialty plants, beverage operations, and seafood and frozen-food plants around the world, seemingly would have no interest in the sales of cigarettes. However, Del Monte is part of the R.J. Reynolds family and thus has a very definite interest in the success of the parent company. Similarly, it is all-in-the-family for Miller beer, with its "father" Philip Morris; and there is a partnership of Saks Fifth Avenue, Gimbels Department Stores, and Brown and Williamson—all members of the Batus family. Some of the family members seem most incompatible. American Brands —makers of Lucky Strikes, Pall Mall, and Tareyton—owns the Franklin Life Insurance Company, which offers discounts on policies to nonsmokers! There is no doubt that, when the tobacco men are feeling pressure (for example, from Congress), they rally the "sibling" companies around the cigarette flag.

Second, tobacco executives know that businesses need clients, and the tobacco empire is a very valuable client, one which businesses in need of accounts would do nothing to displease. Thus, a major chemical company that produces agricultural chemicals is part of the tobacco "family" too, because if it became outspoken on the dangers of cigarettes, it might lose these affluent customers. The roots go even deeper. The suppliers of family companies (glass and container manufacturers for Seven-Up, cans for Miller beer, sugar for Hawaiian Punch, flavoring agents for Patio Mexican foods and Chun King Oriental food) are dealing indirectly, but still significantly, with the tobacco empire.

Third, by teaming up with the manufacturers of other products that might be the subject of bad press or inhibiting government regulation, the cigarette manufacturers are constantly seeking potential allies who will stand by them in the name of Big Business and free enterprise. An analysis of the affiliation of the directors of the top tobacco companies is revealing, as it demonstrates how cigarette manufacturers have been successful in making corporate officers of other industries members of the tobacco team.

Fourth, the cigarette manufacturers demonstrate their economic clout through the use of some of the most elaborate and extravagant advertising and promotional budgets in American history (see section below on the industry's survival strategy). Although they deny publicly that cigarettes are devastating to health, there is no possibility that the decision-makers at the big five tobacco companies are unaware of the risk associated with their product. Thus, they have made a conscious decision that their own economic well-being is far more important than the health of Americans. Advertising is their primary mechanism for neutralizing the medical fears among smokers and keeping the "pleasures" of smoking in the public's mind.

For years, cigarette apologists have defended their advertising practices by claiming that they advertise only to foster competition among various brands, not to mislead smokers about the effects of their habit, or to lure new smokers to the ranks. However, an analysis of the current advertisements for cigarettes strongly suggests that what the ads are selling is not cigarettes, but the *social acceptance of cigarettes*. While smokers today are understandably very nervous and unsure of the legitimacy of their smoking behavior, cigarette advertising reinforces it by giving them reassurance when they need it and communicating that lots of good-looking, healthy, young people smoke.

The heavy reliance on the low-tar and low-nicotine statistics represents an attempt to convey the misleading message that "everything is all right now," but, beyond that, tobacco industry documents reviewed by the FTC indicate that many cigarette advertising techniques are aimed at denigrating or undercutting the health warning. Documents from Brown and Williamson and one of its advertising agencies, Ted Bates and Company, Inc., focused on how to reduce the concern about health effects. As a result of its research, Bates reported to Brown and Williamson that many smokers perceive the habit as "dirty" and dangerous, a practice followed only by "very stupid people." The report concludes:

Thus, the smokers have to face the fact that they are illogical, irrational, and stupid. People find it hard to go throughout life with such negative presentation and evaluation of self. The saviours are the *rationalization* and repression that end up and result in a defense mechanism that, as many of the defense mechanisms we use, has its own logic, its own rationale. [Emphasis theirs.]

The report goes on to recommend that good ad copy will "deemphasize the objections" to smoking. With specific regard to health issues, the Bates report recommends: "Start out from the basic assumption that cigarette smoking is dangerous to your health—try to go around it in an elegant manner but don't try to fight it—it's a losing war."

SELLING DEATH: TOBACCO'S STRATEGY FOR SURVIVAL

For over thirty years, the Office of the Surgeon General has dutifully released reports on the devastating health effects of cigarettes. This year's report focused on the industry's ongoing efforts to entice children to light up. I suggest that next year the Surgeon General take on the most basic of all questions: *How does an industry that sells an inherently dangerous product—lacing it with supplemental nicotine to keep customers addicted—still survive in America in the health conscious 1990s?*

Such a report might begin by shedding light on the tobacco industry's well-orchestrated strategy of providing economic favors, including cold cash, to politicians, the media, social groups, and fellow businessmen in return for their allegiance to its cash cow, the cigarette.

Politicians. We still have, as a book title once put it, "The Best Congress Money Can Buy." Big bucks flow freely to members on both sides of the aisle—and tobacco dollars talk. While one might argue that Congress in the past decade has acted in an increasingly punitive manner toward the cigarette manufacturers, the reality is that the industry has absorbed all the punches and is still quite healthy. Indeed, for the first time in years, statistics indicate that more, not fewer, Americans are smoking. Much of what Congress has done, including banning advertising on TV and radio (the industry actually lobbied for this because they hated the equal time antismoking ads), the prohibition of smoking on airplanes (no real threat to cigarette companies), and the proposed federal tax hike (the industry is expected to "eat" much of it to keep cigarettes affordable) are but annoyances to the merchants of death, all part of the cost of doing business.

Actually Congress remains the number-one protector of the cigarette and will turn deaf ears on any potentially harmful moves against the industry, like the recent proposal to give the FDA control of tobacco products. Most important the Congressional "health" warnings on packs give the industry the most priceless gift: immunity from lawsuits. The label "preempts" industry's responsibility to divulge the specific dangers of its products, and allows the industry's misrepresention campaign (i.e., advertising) to proceed without fear of successful litigation.

Media. Magazines and newspapers in the United States derive much of their revenues from cigarette advertising, guaranteeing editorial silence about the dangers of smoking. Your favorite magazine may cover the "hazards" of processed foods and electric blankets but will spike negative copy about cigarettes.

Social Groups. For many cultural, ethnic, and civic organizations cigarette money is habit forming. For example, the National Women's Political Caucus, the United Negro College Fund, the Gay Men's Health Crisis, universities across the nation (including medical schools)—even the Boy Scouts—are among the unlikely partners in the tobacco business, as they accept donations derived from cigarette sales. It's a good deal for tobacco interests: they get innocence by association and confidence that the very folks who might otherwise express outrage will not join the antismoking chorus.

Tobacco companies own large segments of the food and beverage industry including Kraft-General Foods, Miller Beer (Phillip Morris), and Nabisco and Del Monte (R. J. Reynolds), not to mention a full spectrum of consumer products and services—like Bulova Watches, Jim Beam Bourbon, Loew's Hotels, and Saks Fifth Avenue. Corporate offspring are fiercely loyal to the parent company. Further, cigarette companies are consumers themselves needing chemicals, paper, solvents, and flavoring agents. Thus companies, like Kimberly-Clark (manufacturer of Kleenex, but also the leading provider of cigarette paper) and Borden (distributors of dairy products, but they also make adhesives), become part of the cigarette family, vying to supply, and certainly not alienate, the lucrative cigarette client.

Most recently, tobacco companies have reached out beyond subsidiaries and suppliers to other big-name corporations by offering "free" advertising. In return, a killer industry derives legitimacy from an association with wholesome products. A recent promotional item from Philip Morris, a sleek and feminine "date book," not only glamorizes cigarettes (featuring young women smoking cigarettes while they hail taxi-cabs, paint cars, water gardens, buy health foods, and ride motorbikes), but also carries ads for Cannon Towels, Carnival Cruises, Pfaelzer Brothers steaks, Vidal Sasson, Sunbeam-Oster, Adolfo Luggage, Days Inn, and other top-of-the-line products. Apparently these corporations have no qualms about holding hands in public with tobacco— as long as the advertising is free and effective. Welcome to the extended cigarette family, with all the benefits and obligations that go with it.

By buying its way deep into the nation's political, cultural, and economic fabric, cigarette companies have rendered a remarkable portion of society beholden to and dependent on them. Until the U.S. Congress strips the industry of its privileged legal status, making it face responsibility in court for marketing an inherently hazardous product, and until the industry's current corporate, media, and societal allies divorce themselves from an industry that is literally selling death, the tobacco survival strategy will succeed and the cigarette carnage will continue.

AN UNPRECEDENTED LOBBYING EFFORT

Instead of protecting the public from cigarettes, most tobacco-related laws protect the nicotine industry from being held accountable for their outrageous actions and deadly products. These laws were enacted as a result of the massive political and legislative influence purchased by tobacco companies. The major purpose of their lobbying efforts is to increase or maintain huge profits for the tobacco companies, which means keeping as many people addicted to nicotine as possible.

The tobacco lobby has grown rapidly over the past few

years especially at the state level. During 1991 in California alone, the tobacco industry spent $2.7 million on contributions to politicians. Last year in Pennsylvania more than thirty-five lobbyists worked for the tobacco industry. Such lobbying can effectively block legislation that would decrease smoking rates, reduce the sale of cigarettes to minors, and protect nonsmokers from passive smoke in public places.

Lobbying has kept vending-machine sales of cigarettes alive. Many studies have documented how easily children can buy cigarettes through vending machines. One survey commissioned by National Automatic Merchandizing Association (NAMA) found that thirteen-year-olds were eleven times more likely than were seventeen-year-olds to buy cigarettes from the machines. Although less than one percent of adult smokers buy cigarettes primarily from vending machines, there are more than 600,000 of these mechanical drug dealers in America, accounting for more than half of all locations where cigarettes are sold.

Pro-health activists have lobbied to enact more than 140 local ordinances in the past three years that eliminate or restrict the placement of cigarette vending machines. Vending-machine companies have joined with the tobacco lobby in opposing the ordinances. Lawsuits have even been filed to strike down these local laws. None of these court challenges, however, has yet succeeded.

The tobacco lobby is also trying to get state statutes enacted that would preempt (outlaw) all local cigarette vending-machine ordinances. In order to succeed, tobacco lobbyists have been drafting and promoting state legislation that deceptively appears to protect minors from illegal vending-machine sales. But careful analysis of the wording in these bills reveals that few, if any, vending machines would be eliminated and that only those who profit from illegal cigarette sales would receive any type of protection.

In an effort to immunize themselves from lawsuits by tobacco victims, tobacco companies have been spending much time and money lobbying for product-liability reform. Any successful litigation would encourage an onslaught of similar suits and force manufacturers finally to be legally accountable for their deadly products and egregious actions. Manufacturers would then be forced to raise cigarette prices substantially to cover plaintiff awards and court costs. Like tax increases, these price hikes would further reduce the nicotine addiction rate.

In lobbying for product liability legislation, the tobacco companies have organized powerful coalitions with multinational manufacturers of other products. For public-relations purposes, these coalitions claim that they want to reduce frivolous lawsuits against small local employers, who are given token status in the coalitions.

The tobacco industry reacts to local attempts to ban public smoking by greatly expanding its lobbying presence at the state level. In 1988 and 1989 the industry successfully lobbied half a dozen state legislatures, including Florida, Pennsylvania, and Illinois, to enact statutes that specifically preempt local laws, but provide little or no protection from tobacco smoke. Although the tobacco lobby publicly claimed to oppose these so-called state indoor-air laws, the tobacco industry was their only beneficiary.

Recognizing that state indoor-air laws that preempt local laws rarely promote health, pro-health activists have successfully prevented their enactment in other states. Non-preemptive clean-indoor-air laws have also been enacted at the state level, but most of these provide very little protection from tobacco smoke. In fact, at the state level, most of the laws that affect tobacco protect the industry.

Coping with Disaster

The complexity of the cigarette's ongoing devastation to public health in America sometimes appears overwhelming as it becomes enmeshed with human frailties. The dominant cigarette industry, together with its associated subindustries, is unequivocally committed to serving the needs of that human frailty, no matter what the cost. However, there are a number of specific courses this country could take to cope with the national health disaster created by cigarette smoking.

First and foremost, before we as a country can begin a plan of action to deal with the cigarette, we must face up to the enormity of the problem that cigarettes now pose. We have to cast aside that sense of resignation to cigarettes and death and recognize cigarettes for what they are—a unique problem that merits a unique solution.

One might initially be tempted to argue that cigarettes are not any different from alcohol or even food, that anything can be overused to the point of becoming a health threat. Actually, unlike other forms of legal recreation such as alcohol consumption, there is, for all practical purposes, no known safe level of cigarette use, nor any known health benefit. While there are those who abuse alcohol, either by drinking to the point where it becomes physically damaging or combining drinking with driving an automobile, the majority of people who use alcohol consume it at levels that are harmless. (There is even evidence that moderate alcohol consumption may confer some protection against heart disease.) The overwhelming majority of smokers, however, smoke at levels definitely detrimental to health. Due to their addictive nature, it is for all practical purposes not possible to smoke a "safe" number of cigarettes per day.

Let us, as a country, make a policy decision one way or another on cigarettes. Given our experiences with Prohibition in the 1920s, when the government attempted to deny access to a commodity that people wanted, the outlawing of cigarettes seems like an unrealistic option. However, we can remove our heads from the sand and face the ultimate question: Are the economic benefits of cigarettes important enough to this country that they justify the premature deaths of 500,000 Americans each year, as well as the tens of billion of dollars it costs to treat the resultant health disasters and make up for lost productivity?

Even if the answer is yes, do we choose to continue to disperse the enormous costs of smoking throughout the entire population and, indeed, to subsidize the production of tobacco? Or will we adopt the policy of letting people smoke cigarettes as they please, but no longer make the nonsmoking population foot the bill in terms of the costs of extensive medical care, lost workdays, fire damage, and increased life-insurance costs?

Were we to face up to these questions and familiarize American nonsmokers with the enormous amounts of money they are paying for the smoker's "right" to light up, we might have one of the answers to the cigarette dilemma in America—let those who wish to smoke do so, but also let the smokers and companies that market cigarettes assume all the economic responsibilities of the habit.

Second, both voluntary and government agencies should

escalate their attempts to bring warnings on the danger of smoking both to smokers and nonsmokers. In waging his war against more detailed cigarette health warnings, Sen. Wendell H. Ford (D.Ky.) maintained that there was an "exceptionally high level of awareness" on the issue of smoking and the American public is "bombarded with information on smoking." Indeed a superficial look at recent Roper and Gallup polls seems to back him up, given that 90 percent of those surveyed knew that smoking could be "dangerous." However, the more-in-depth questions in these surveys noted that 30 percent of Americans were unaware that a thirty-year-old man reduces his life expectancy by smoking a pack a day; 43 percent were unaware that smoking is a major cause of heart disease; and up to 80 percent of the population did not know that smoking causes most bronchitis and emphysema. Many anecdotal accounts from physicians indicate that nearly every patient who receives a diagnosis of lung cancer is shocked, angry, and indignant, claiming that he or she just didn't know that "only" a pack a day would cause this disease.

Third, we could give some serious consideration to whether our society should encourage the production of increasingly brazen tobacco advertisements, which associate smoking with glamour, youth, and good clean fun. It might be argued that cigarette advertisements perform a function by providing tar and nicotine levels, but this could be done without the Satin Doll, the macho cowboy, and the athlete putting his socks on in the locker room. Toning down the ads, and perhaps eliminating them entirely except at point of purchase, might have the additional benefit of removing the editorial hesitancy to cover the topic of cigarettes in popular magazines.

Fourth, the concept of cigarette addiction needs more attention than it has received. The nicotine patch, when used in conjunction with behavior modification classes, has shown promise in breaking this addiction. Further efforts along this line are desperately needed.

The cigarette has been maligned by a series of critics through the ages, but, until thirty years ago, the attacks were primarily emotional, with heavy moral overtones. In the 1990s we should not be moralizing about cigarettes, but simply facing up to the realities and asking ourselves, if we really want to win the war against environmental disease, why don't we start by identifying the number-one enemy?

Suggestions for the Future

January 11, 1994, marked the thirtieth anniversary of the release of the first surgeon general's report linking cigarette smoking and disease. The 1964 official government report (which could have been released ten years earlier as the data were available then) triggered a cascade of events aimed at discouraging smoking.

Thirty years later, with more than 25 percent of Americans still regularly smoking cigarettes, with a substantial number of recent surveys indicating that smoking is again on the rise, and with a staggering annual cigarette-induced death toll of 500,000, it is time to acknowledge that our current policies to curb smoking simply are not working. On this thirtieth anniversary, the U.S. Congress should order the formation of a new commission—one that considers more innovative and effective approaches to solving our nation's pandemic of cigarette-related disease.

I propose here one modest yet potentially extremely effective new strategy which the new commission should consider: *removing the government warning label currently on cigarette packages.*

The warning labels, while presumably well intentioned, have done nothing to discourage smoking, but have provided extraordinary legal protection for the industry such that this killer product still thrives today.

During the mid-1960s, when the health hazards of smoking finally became undeniable to policy makers (the dangers were obvious to the scientific community by the late 1930s), both public health activists and the tobacco industry lobbied Congress for warning labels. Health advocates thought they were "doing good." The industry acted to ensure survival: as more states proposed different warning statements on packs, the potential for chaos in interstate commerce was a looming nightmare. Better to have just one, standard label, they reasoned. But via this government action, the industry sought more: immunity from all the lawsuits which inevitably would be brought by smokers who would become ill and die from smoking cigarettes. As a direct result of the 1965 congressionally mandated "health" label (which was extended to include advertisements in 1969), the industry was given a unique and privileged legal status, a teflon coating which repelled all liability claims. Whether this windfall for the industry was an inadvertent result of well-meaning government action or was the product of industry manipulation of Congress is a matter of historical debate. But the end result was that industry attorneys for years have used a non-sequitur defense arguing that, in essence, "cigarettes are not dangerous, but if they are, which they are not, the government 'preempted' our responsiblity to warn of those dangers." Put another way, the industry is saying "Gee, we would like to tell you folks more details about the health risks of smoking, but the government took this authority away from us when they mandated a label, so don't blame us now for not warning sufficiently." The U.S. Supreme Court in 1992 largely agreed that the government warning label preempted lawsuits, although it did leave a window open if an industry disinformation conspiracy could be established.

The threat of litigation is a clear and powerful incentive for an industry to keep its product safe, or to be very, very specific about the dangers associated with its use. Given its Congressionally bestowed litigation shield (the industry has never paid a cent in damages), cigarette manufacturers have no incentive whatever to be honest about the consequences of smoking and have apparently unlimited freedom to distort, misrepresent, and maim.

For example:

- Despite 60,000 medical citations to the contrary, industry spokesmen continue to maintain that there is *no* evidence that smoking adversely affects health. In November 1993 during sworn testimony in a Miami trial, Michael Rosenbaum, Vice President of the holding company that owns Liggett Group Inc. (Chesterfield, L&M, and other brands), when asked if cigarettes cause cancer, responded evasively, "I'm not a medical doctor. I don't have a clue." Lorillard's Andrew Tisch, when queried about smoking causing disease, also demured: "If it turns out that's true, I will be very upset."

- Tobacco companies spend $4 billion annually to promote cigarettes as healthy, invigorating, and generally part of the good life, a clear distortion of the grim medical realities. Only an industry that perceives itself as immune from lawsuits would have the gall to offer "free" designer clothing (Virginia Slims attire, fashions any young woman would just die for) in return for proof of purchase of 975 packs of cigarettes in a six-month period—a consumption rate in excess of five packs per day. (Would a liquor company get away with enticing consumers to purchase 5 fifths of alcohol a day?)

Advocates for tobacco control frequently contend that the solution to our nation's pandemic of cigarette-related diseases—now accounting for one in four deaths annually—is *more* government intervention: a ban on advertising, a hike in the excise tax, and restrictions on smoking in public places.

But the truth is that if government had not meddled in the first place, the "system" would have worked. Cigarette companies would have conducted business on the same legal turf as every other industry. They would have been sued by smokers or the families of smokers who suffered and died prematurely. And the industry would have been assessed damages because they marketed an inherently hazardous product without full disclosure. Cigarette advertising would long ago have been voluntarily withdrawn by the industry (it would be incompatible with any defense in court), and the price of cigarettes would have soared (without a bureaucratically inspired "sin-tax") as the increased costs were passed on to smokers. If Congress had not legislated the label and the legal immunity it spawned, cigarettes might still be available, but the industry would be totally forthright about risks and might even require written, informed consent from the smoker as a means of protecting itself against further liability. If free market forces and an unfettered judicial system had prevailed, the cigarette would now be an anachronism simply because it would be too expensive to buy and too unprofitable to produce. Thirty years after proof of cause was established, let's get serious about making the cigarette industry accountable for its actions: Remove the government warning label now.

How to Reduce Your Risks of Cancer

To avoid tobacco-related diseases and death, *don't start smoking*. If you do smoke, *quit*. Tell your children, friends, colleagues not to smoke or use any other form of tobacco.

4

Alcohol

There is clear evidence that excessive alcohol consumption increases the risk of specific cancers, especially in connection with cigarette smoking—specifically, esophageal, oral, pharyngeal, laryngeal, and liver cancers. People who smoke *and* drink have an even higher rate than do people who smoke *or* drink.

The alcohol-cancer association was first suspected some time around the turn of the century, when it was noticed that men who worked at jobs where heavy alcohol consumption was encouraged developed cancer more often than people not employed in these professions. A recent study in Denmark showed that brewery workers have a higher risk of cancer than does the general population. In 1979 a study in Denmark revealed that according to traditional practice in various breweries, employees received approximately four liters of free beer each day as an employee "perk." Presumably, the beer was consumed, resulting in a greater-than-average consumption of beer among brewery workers. Accordingly,

153

they had a greater-than-expected number of cancer deaths from esophageal, laryngeal, lung, and liver cancer. Other evidence suggests that heavy alcohol consumption, sufficient to cause cirrhosis of the liver, also increases the incidence of liver cancer.

In contrast, populations who traditionally abstain from alcohol (for example, the Mormons) have very low rates of cancer in these sites.

Alcoholic beverages have been consumed by humans for at least five thousand years. Only recently, though, has the alcohol in these drinks been suspected of being a carcinogen. Information on the subject of alcohol and cancer is still incomplete because the whole subject is very new. For example, the American Cancer Society's book *Cancer: A Manual for Practitioners*, which was published in 1970, doesn't even mention that alcohol may play a role in cancer causation. Similarly, the *Special Report to Congress on Alcohol and Health*, published by the Public Health Service in 1971, never mentioned cancer (the second report, put out in 1974, however, did).

From the start, the association between spirit consumption and malignant disease was difficult to establish. Animal studies are not very helpful. Even at high-dose levels (20 percent pure alcohol in drinking water given for long periods of time), it does not cause a tumor increase in animals. It seems that pure alcohol is not in itself carcinogenic to laboratory animals.

Studies of human drinking habits have been thwarted repeatedly because people tend not to "remember" how much they really drink. Unless you measure your intake very carefully, your response would only be a rough estimate. And if you drink a lot, your estimate would probably be on the low side. Beyond that, the harmful effects of alcohol and cigarette smoke are so closely entwined (one study of alcoholics showed that 94 percent of them smoked) that it is usually difficult to tell which factor is really responsible for the cancer that develops.

Adding to the confusion are strong personal convictions about the morality, or lack thereof, of drinking. Teetotaling researchers might feel a little differently from those who enjoy a nightly cocktail hour. Similar to the case for cigarettes, research on alcohol has been somewhat shortchanged because of our society's extreme fondness for wine, beer, and distilled liquors. Perhaps it is only human nature to ignore information that implies something you like is harmful.

Much effort has gone into trying to find out if the association between alcohol and cancer is due to the alcohol itself or to other chemicals that are found in alcoholic beverages. Some evidence suggests that the effect is greatest in distilled liquors, and some other evidence shows that the apple-based drinks (such as apple cider) used in northern France are particularly potent cancer-causers. Most of the evidence in humans, however, suggests that carcinogenesis is related to the alcohol itself, rather than the substances specific to the form in which it is drunk.

Still another hypothesis is that alcohol acts as a cocarcinogen (that means two substances act together to cause cancer). This is supported by several studies showing that among nonsmokers, heavy alcohol consumption is associated with just two or three times the rate of oral, pharyngeal, and esophageal cancers. In smokers, however, consumption of the same amount of alcohol is associated with much higher cancer levels in these sites. Alcohol and tobacco together have far more than an additive effect on such cancers.

How Much Is Too Much?

Definitions of "heavy" drinking vary, but generally speaking most scientific studies draw the line at two or three ounces of absolute alcohol a day.

If you drink more than three ounces of alcohol each day—roughly the equivalent of three drinks each made with two ounces of eighty-proof liquor; five five-ounce glasses of wine; or six eight-ounce glasses of beer—you would be considered a heavy drinker. If you did not drink every day but went on "binges" that averaged out to that daily level, you would also be considered a heavy drinker.

However, the relationship between alcohol consumption and cancer is not a clearcut dose-response situation, where increasing the amount drunk increases the likelihood of getting cancer proportionally. So, if you had four drinks a day, you would not necessarily have X times the cancer risk of somebody who consumed fewer drinks per day.

The Health Benefits of Moderate Alcohol Consumption

Data from epidemiologic studies within recent decades demonstrate that death rates from coronary heart disease are lower among consumers of small to moderate amounts of alcohol than among nondrinkers. Some of the proposed mechanisms for the beneficial health effects of moderate alcohol consumption are:

- alcohol lowers harmful LDL-cholesterol levels;

- alcohol raises protective HDL-cholesterol levels;

- alcohol decreases formation of blood clots in the arteries;

- alcohol increases coronary blood flow;

- alcohol increases estrogen levels.

At low to moderate levels of intake the adverse effects do not outweigh the beneficial effects, in regard to the mortality from coronary heart disease. Thus, the net effect of the reported consumption of small to moderate amounts of alcohol is a reduction of the total mortality of the drinking population.

What Types of Cancer Are Associated with Alcohol Consumption?

Cancers at those sites related to alcohol consumption (oral, pharyngeal, esophageal, laryngeal, and liver) account for 6.5 percent of all cancer deaths and 6 percent of all cancer cases, but this proportion probably overlaps considerably with the cancer cases and deaths attributable to tobacco smoking.

THE ESOPHAGUS

The risk of esophageal cancer is many times greater among alcoholics than among nondrinkers and even among lighter drinkers, with estimates ranging from eleven to eighteen times higher. The greater the alcohol consumption, the higher the risk of esophageal cancer. A French study found that the risk for people who drank less than one ounce of alcohol per day was not elevated over the normal risk, whereas people who drank two ounces per day tripled their risk; for those who consumed more than three ounces, there was an eighteenfold increase.

In addition, smoking greatly enhances the cancer risk. People who smoke and drink have more than an additive effect—they have a multiplicative effect. In simplistic terms, if drinking increased your risk by five times and smoking by five times independent of that risk, your risk would not be 5 + 5, or 10, but rather 5 × 5, or 25 times greater. But, even in the absence of smoking, the risk of esophageal cancer for drinkers is very high.

There has been some evidence that the type of alcohol influences esophageal cancer risk. Risks tend to be somewhat higher for drinkers of hard liquor than for regular consumers of beer or wine, but rising trends in risk are noted with increasing consumption in each category.

In many parts of the world, select alcoholic beverages are linked to unusually high risks for esophageal cancer. In Africa, for example, home-made brews are associated with this form of cancer. A Chinese liquor made with rice and some grain alcohol (either barley, maize, or wheat) also poses a higher risk, as does a distilled spirit made of southern Brazil from sugar cane (Cachaca) and a Puerto Rican home-brewed rum. This suggests that, in addition to ethanol, some other ingredient in certain alcoholic beverages plays a role in causing cancer.

ORAL CANCER

Alcohol and tobacco are both risk factors for cancer of the mouth and pharynx; together they are thought to be responsible for about 75 percent of all cancers of the oral cavity in American men. It is particularly difficult to sort out the effects of tobacco smoke and alcohol on oral cancers. A few studies have looked at oral cancer while controlling for cigarette smoking and have shown that heavy drinkers that do not smoke increase their risk of oral cancer by two or three times. Certainly this would be much higher for heavy smokers.

CANCER OF THE LARYNX

Laryngeal cancer is much more common among alcoholics than among nonalcoholics. Part of this increase may be due to the effects of cigarette smoking, but certainly not all. The rates of laryngeal cancer are known to rise with increasing alcohol intake in lifelong nonsmokers, confirming that smoking is not a prerequisite. Again, a working "risk factor" of two or three times greater risk of laryngeal cancer may apply here. In some countries of southwest Europe, including Spain, France, and Italy, the incidence of laryngeal cancer is very high, possibly related to excessive wine consumption.

LIVER CANCER

Alcoholics with cirrhosis of the liver, or alcohol-induced liver damage, have a much higher than average rate of liver cancer. On autopsy an estimated 60 to 90 percent of patients with primary liver cancer also have cirrhosis. Additional studies, however, have found liver cancer in the absence of cirrhosis. Whether or not this has any relevance to moderate drinkers is not known. Because the liver is the organ that detoxifies potentially cancer-causing substances in the body, it seems at least possible that constant, massive amounts of alcohol may damage the liver sufficiently to set the stage for carcinogenic growth. No evidence yet exists that moderate drinkers, or even heavy drinkers who are not alcoholics, are likely to suffer higher than the average risk of getting liver cancer. Perhaps this is because liver cancer is a fairly rare disease in our country.

BREAST CANCER

There have been conflicting reports about alcohol consumption and breast cancer. Certain studies indicate that the risk of breast cancer in women may increase with only moderate levels of alcohol intake. For example, data from the Nurses' Health Study indicate that in comparison with women who stated that they consumed alcohol, those who consumed three to nine drinks per week had a 30 percent increased risk of having breast cancer. Those who drank more than nine drinks had a 60 percent increased risk over nondrinkers.

Other studies indicate no such relation between moderate alcohol intake and increased risk of breast cancer. For example, the Framingham Study did not find an increase in breast cancer rates among women who consumed small to moderate amounts of alcohol. In addition, in nations where wine consumption (as well as total alcohol consumption) is highest, breast cancer rates are not higher than those in countries with low alcohol consumption. Age-standardized death rates for breast cancer among women, as reported by the World Health Organization for 1987, were 28, 29, and 21 per 100,000 from three countries with the most wine consumption—France, Italy, and Spain, respectively. For three countries with very low wine consumption, the U.S., Great Britain and Ireland, they were 32, 41 and 38, respectively. However, these cultural comparisons do not provide enough evidence to conclude that alcohol does not affect breast cancer rates. Other lifestyle factors in the countries with a high intake of wine could ameliorate the effect of alcohol. It will require further research to clearly define what role, if any, alcohol plays in breast cancer.

OTHER CANCERS

There is no firm evidence to suggest that alcohol consumption increases your risk of getting any other types of cancer, although several investigations have looked into cancers at other sites, including the stomach, colon, rectum, pancreas, and bladder. Research continues on these issues.

How Alcohol Might Increase Your Cancer Risk

DIET

People who drink large amounts of alcohol can become poorly nourished for two reasons. First, they eat fewer of the nutrients needed to stay healthy (simply because they aren't hungry after drinking so much). Among heavy drinkers, the percentage of calories derived from alcohol can be quite substantial. One survey found that people who consumed the equivalent of about 2.5 or more drinks per day got about one-quarter of their daily calories from alcohol alone. This survey found that intake of protein and several vitamins, especially A and C, was significantly decreased. A multitude of studies has found the alcoholic's intake of thiamine, folic acid, magnesium, iron, and zinc to be severely diminished. Second, alcohol may impair the body's ability to absorb the nutrients that are taken in.

Scientists believe that this double-faceted nutrient deficiency predisposes people to the carcinogenic effects of alcohol. This may be because tissues that are lacking in nutrients may not be able to stand up to the chemical wear and tear of alcohol.

TISSUE CHANGES

The type of cancers most commonly associated with frequent consumption of alcoholic beverages are those of the tissues in contact with the alcohol as it enters the body. These are the mouth, esophagus, larynx, stomach, and liver (through which alcohol absorbed in the stomach first passes before entering the general circulation). For example, smokers who drink have a much higher rate of esophageal cancer than smokers who don't drink, but both groups have similar rates of lung cancer. This pattern of behavior—increasing the risk at points of entry into the body—is often seen with locally acting carcinogens.

Alcohol is an irritant to living tissues. Repeated contact with concentrated alcohol solutions could produce in the tissues of the mouth, esophagus, liver, etc. a variety of irritant effects which are known to "promote" the development of cancer. Other body sites come in contact with alcohol after it has been diluted by the body water and this should be affected to a much smaller degree, if at all. Irritation *per se* is not believed to cause cancer but it is known to enhance the effects of direct-acting carcinogens. These are agents that actually can convert a normal cell into a cancerous cell. To do this, however, direct-acting carcinogens require help from substances called "promoters." These promoters are generally substances which irritate cells or otherwise disrupt the normal communication between cells in tissues. By stimulating cells to multiply, promoters appear to allow cells to permanently "lock in" the genetic damage that seems to convert normal cells to cancer cells and to allow the new cancer cells to get a good start toward growing into a clinically detectable tumor.

In a crude sense, you can think of the effects of promoters on potential cancer cells as being similar to the effect of fertilizing on the growth of your garden. The overall effect of promoters in human cancer may be very significant. For example, studies show that smokers have a twenty-to-thirty times greater risk of lung cancer than nonsmokers. People who stop smoking, however, very rapidly begin to decrease their risk of lung cancer. This risk drops to less than half of that seen in smokers by five years after a person quits smoking. The risk continues to decline, settling down eventually to only about double over that among those who never smoked. Most scientists attribute this large and rapid decrease in risk in ex-smokers to the effect of stopping daily exposure to the cancer-promoting substances in tobacco smoke. As we already discussed, alcohol is known to increase the risk of esophageal cancer in smokers from eighteen- to fifty-fold. Scientists generally attribute this to the "promoting" effects of alcohol.

Alcohol also decreases saliva and mucous flow in the mouth and esophagus. This may leave the delicate membranes of the mouth and esophagus exposed to more direct access by various direct carcinogens. Alcoholic beverages contain a variety of amines, aldehydes, and ketones that may also play a role.

SUPPRESS IMMUNE FUNCTION

Alcoholics frequently have impaired immune functions. The ability of the immune system to attack and destroy early cancer appears to play a role in the body's natural defenses against cancer. As mentioned before, the damage to the liver seen in chronic alcoholics may also hamper the functioning of the liver enzymes which normally detoxify a variety of potential cancer-causing substances—both those produced within the body and those taken into the body.

COCARCINOGENS

There is good reason to believe that alcohol, instead of acting by itself to cause cancers, is a "cocarcinogen"—that is, it promotes cancer in combination with another "direct" car-cinogen. The most serious and common example we have of this is alcohol consumption combined with cigarette smok-ing, which greatly increases the risk of cancer. If you smoke two packs of cigarettes a day, you assume a 143 percent greater risk of developing cancer of the oral cavity than does a person who doesn't smoke. If, in addition to this you have just two alcoholic drinks per day, your risk increases to almost 1500 percent. Scientists believe that alcohol multiplies the effects of tobacco smoke at other sites, as well, especially the esophagus and larynx, but probably not the lung (since alcohol does not come into contact with that organ).

How Important Is the Risk of Getting Cancer from Alcohol in Comparison to Other Causes of Cancer?

How important the risk is depends on how much you drink and your other habits. The more moderate your consumption, the smaller the risk. If you smoke, you shouldn't drink at all. And even though heavy drinking in itself may not significantly increase your risk of cancer, there are plenty of other good reasons to moderate alcohol use. Heavy drinking is simply not worth the risks it carries with it—not just increased cancer risks, but its role in liver ailments and other diseases. Alcohol can contribute to obesity, too, since it is an extremely dense source of calories. But, on the other hand, we have to put some kind of perspective on the risk of getting cancer from alcohol consumption.

In 1985, around 250,000 American men died of cancer, and some 90 percent of these cancers occurred at sites with no apparent link with alcohol. If as much as half of the rest of these deaths were associated with alcohol consumption, that would mean that all but 12,500 cancer deaths were related to alcohol consumption—about 4 percent of all cancer deaths for that year. This is a rather small percentage in contrast to cigarette-induced cancer, which alone accounted for over 30 percent of all male cancer deaths that same year. The increasing, and justified, public health action against alcohol abuse should be based on its other adverse effects, not for its role in cancer causation.

Alcohol Is Alcohol

Recently, American preferences for alcohol have taken a turn toward "light" alcoholic beverages. White wine, light beer, vodka, and white rum have replaced some of the more traditional "heavy" drinks such as martinis and manhattans. Much of this shift seems to be driven by diet consciousness. White wine and light beer do contain fewer calories per ounce than distilled spirits. Part of the change in preference may also be tied to negative images associated by many with "booze."

In discussing alcohol as a possible cancer-causing agent, it is important to recognize that how much you drink (in terms of total alcohol) is far more important than what form you drink the alcohol in. There has been some speculation about the nonalcoholic constituents of beer, wine, and distilled spirits and their effect on cancer causation over and above the alcohol itself. Some evidence has suggested that the effect is most significant when alcohol is consumed in "hard" form (80 proof and greater). Others have suggested that apple-based liquor consumed in Northwest France is particularly harmful. But the totality of evidence suggests that it is *alcohol,* from any source in any form, that plays a role either directly in cancer causation or as a cocarcinogen.

The confusion arises because many people make a mental distinction between beer and wine, on the one hand, and "hard liquor" or booze on the other. Just consider how many local governments apply controls to the sale of beer and wine that are different from those applied to the sale of liquor. There is a tendency in the popular mind to associate the ill effects of excessive drinking only with booze. Scientifically, however, alcohol is alcohol. You can drink too much beer or wine just as you can drink too much liquor.

Either way, the risk of various health problems is increased, including cancer. It all depends on how much you drink.

The alcoholic content of distilled spirits like gin, bourbon, whisky, scotch, and vodka is expressed in terms of the proof. The proof of the liquor is twice the alcohol content—so an 80 proof bottle of Scotch is 40 percent alcohol. Table wines contain about 12 percent alcohol. Although there may be slight variations according to the type of grape used, and variation in soil or climate during the growing season, basically there seems to be no difference between the physiological effects or alcoholic contents of red and white wines. Red wines are made by fermenting grape juice with the skins added in; white wine is made by fermenting grape juice without grape skins. As a result, red wines are richer in pigmented compounds and tannins than white wines, but the alcohol content (most important as a cancer risk factor) of table wines is relatively constant at about 12 percent.

Fortified wines, on the other hand, have an alcoholic content of about 20 percent by volume. The extra alcohol is usually derived from neutral spirits made from wine or brandy. Liqueurs vary in alcoholic content from 20 to 55 percent. And beer contains 3 to 6 percent alcohol (large beer) or 4 to 8 percent (stout).

If we were to compare three glasses of wine to a martini (assuming that the martini contained about 3 ounces with a 7.1 ratio of gin to vermouth) we would find that: 15 ounces of wine × 12 percent alcohol is 1.8 ounces of pure alcohol; 2.6 ounces of gin × 40 percent alcohol plus 0.4 ounces of vermouth at 20 percent alcohol equals 1.1 ounces of pure alcohol. Obviously, "light drinkers" who drink only wine can easily consume more alcohol than their compatriots drinking the hard stuff.

Alcohol, Nutrition, and Cancer

If you drink regularly, you should keep in mind that each gram of alcohol that the body takes in yields seven calories. That means that five ounces of wine yields 90 to 100 calories, a martini 220, an ounce of eighty-proof Scotch 80, and a twelve-ounce can of beer around 170.

Even a moderate drinker can quickly accumulate many unnecessary calories, and since these calories do not contain significant amounts of required nutrients, nutrition can become borderline or poor if drinking replaces eating. For example, if you have two martinis at lunch, two before dinner and a glass of wine with dinner, you are consuming not only more than five ounces of pure alcohol, but also nearly 1,000 empty calories. Even if you are following a very liberal daily caloric intake of 3,000 a day, alcohol will account for one-third of your total calories. Again, it might be easy to cut back by skimping on food, and "drinking your lunch," even if this involves, for the sake of propriety, ordering a meal and then just not eating very much of it.

Is There a Safe Limit?

Clearly there is a great deal to be learned about the effects of various levels of alcohol consumption on cancer risk. We really do not know at this point how much is too much. Certainly individual susceptibility to alcohol-related problems—especially alcoholism—is a critical factor.

If calories are a source of concern, that reason alone is enough to be moderate about drinking, be it cocktails, beer, or wine. Beyond that, a rule of thumb, supported by extensive epidemiological data, is to limit alcohol consumption to one to two drinks per day. A drink is defined as ten to twelve grams of ethyl alcohol, which is approximately equivalent to one twelve-ounce can or bottle of beer, four to five ounces of table wine or 1.25 ounces of eighty-proof spirits.

How to Reduce Your Risk of Cancer

1. If you do choose to drink each day, turn down the third one. Two per day is enough. Skip the drinks at lunch. Keep your intake of alcoholic beverages below 2.5 ounces of eighty-proof liquor, two five-ounce glasses of wine, or two twelve-ounce cans of beer.

2. If you must smoke even a few cigarettes a day (although it would be better not to smoke at all!), *do not make things any worse* by consuming alcohol, even if you are drinking at a time when you're not smoking.

3. If you do drink each day, make sure your alcohol intake does not interfere with your eating a well-balanced meal. In particular, be sure you get enough food with B vitamins and iron, particularly whole-grain products, green leafy vegetables, corn, nuts, potatoes, fruits such as raisins, grapes, and peaches, and, occasionally, liver.

5

Sunlight

Throughout much of Western history, fair skin has been considered a desirable feature, at least until relatively recently. Marie Antoinette's complexion was described as "an appealing blend of lilies and roses." In the seventeenth and eighteenth centuries, French women are said to have put leeches on their faces to reduce the blood supply brought to their faces. In Georgian England, women painted themselves with a white lead mixture—the mark of a lady was her enchanting, pale complexion.

On the other hand, a tanned and weather-beaten complexion used to be traditionally associated with the lower classes, for both men and women. There are people still living who recall when women did not leave the house in sunny weather without a hat or parasol.

Although in some ancient cultures the sun was worshipped as a god, the use of the sun was limited to religious or specific therapeutic purposes. Before the twentieth century, examples of white-skinned people voluntarily expos-

171

ing themselves to the sun for prolonged periods of time were extremely rare. And so was the incidence of skin cancer.

In 1896, Dr. Paul Unna described a disease he called "seamanshaut" because he saw it particularly often in sailors. Within the next ten years, other researchers reported cases of what they termed "tropical skin" among outdoor laborers. In 1920, Dr. James McCoy wrote in the *Archives of Dermatology and Syphilology,* "The face, neck and hands comprise but a small surface of the body, yet according to my personal observations 49.6 percent of all cancers are cutaneous cancers of these parts."

These reports were but of passing interest to most people, since Americans were not in the habit of toasting themselves in the sun. Everyone wore long-sleeved clothing and hats, which protected them from the sun's ultraviolet rays. When they did go to the beach, they wore modest and very heavy bathing costumes, and sat in protected areas.

Things began to change in the 1930s when it became the fashion for women to show "more skin," and clothing became lighter. People had more leisure time and spent more time at the beach. Suddenly, "tan was beautiful." By the 1940s, both men and women were spending summer days soaking up rays and sometimes even encouraging a sunburn by using reflectors or covering themselves with oil. Wealthy people maintained year-round tans by vacationing in the south.

By the 1950s, the incidence of skin cancer had increased significantly. In the 1990s, this formerly rare disease is the most diagnosed of all cancers in the United States, accounting for 39 percent of all diagnosed malignancies.

A great deal of evidence points to the sun's ultraviolet rays as the prime cause of skin cancer. Those races with pigmented skin have skin cancer rates far lower than those of light-skinned populations. More than 90 percent of skin cancers occur on areas of the body not protected by clothing, such as the face, ears, neck, lower lip, and back of the hands. Skin cancer is also much more common in tropical and subtropical areas than it is where the sun is not so intense on a year-round basis. The nonmelanoma skin cancer rate doubles every five hundred to seven hundred miles as one approaches the equator. Fishermen, farmers, professional athletes, and those who work outdoors get skin cancer much more frequently than do people whose occupations keep them indoors. Frequent exposure to ultraviolet rays will induce skin cancer in laboratory animals, too. Ninety percent of nonmelanoma skin cancers are linked with exposure to sunlight, as are 50 percent or more of melanomas.

Skin Basics

Skin is multilayered. The outer layers comprise the epidermis, the middle layers the dermis, and innermost are the subcutaneous layers. The outer layer of the epidermis, the keratin layer, contains a substance known as melanin, a dense and insoluble material that is so durable that it persists in the skin of mummies. Enough melanin in the skin prevents the penetration of ultraviolet rays to underlying and sensitive layers of the skin. Blacks have a great deal of melanin; albinos have none.

When you are exposed to the sun, the first result is a slight tan, which is caused by the darkening of whatever melanin is already present in your skin. Even if you have very little melanin and expose yourself for only a small amount of time, the melanin present in your skin will be able to protect you. If the melanin is distributed unevenly through your skin, you'll get freckles. No matter how much melanin your skin contains, if you get too much sun, cells on the top layers will die and allow ultraviolet rays to penetrate to deeper tissues. This can result in cellular changes and slowing of growth in nearby cells. If these changes occur often enough, they may set the stage for the development of malignant skin tumors later in life. If you continue to bask in the sun, especially if you have fair skin, you are inviting skin cancer.

Teenage girls seem to be the most difficult group to convince about the dangers of the sun. To them, "tan is beautiful," and age fifty-five seems a long way off. Most dermatologists now think that exposure to excessive amounts of intense sunlight during the teen years starts the cancer process in skin tissue. Continued exposure in the twenties, thirties, and later makes the situation even worse. But skin is most sensitive in individuals under the age of twenty.

This doesn't mean you should avoid the sun completely. Even dermatologists who offer the grimmest warnings on the dangers of the sun concede that there are circumstances where exposure to the sun's rays can be helpful. The summer sun often relieves asthma, aching joints, psoriasis, and acne. A day on the beach can also be an enjoyable experience for most of us. The key here is knowing when you've had enough and to use appropriate protection, such as cover-up clothing, umbrellas, and sunscreens.

Skin Cancer: Not Just One Cancer

There are approximately three-quarters of a million cases of skin cancer diagnosed every year in this country, making it the most common form of cancer today. Three types of skin cancer account for the majority of malignant skin tumors: basal cell, squamous cell, and melanoma.

BASAL CELL CANCER

About three-quarters of all skin cancers are basal cell. Previously considered a condition of people older than forty, basal cell cancers are afflicting increasing numbers of young people. The primary reason: excess sun exposure. Basal cell cancers generally occur on the face and ears, and are so named because they occur in the layer of cells that forms the base of the epidermis. Although basal cell cancer is slow growing and generally doesn't spread to distant parts of the body, it needs to be treated promptly and thoroughly. Left untreated, basal cell cancers can spread and invade bone and underlying tissue. Once treated, people who have had this type of cancer should vigilantly check for further cancers, as there is a significant chance of recurrence.

SQUAMOUS CELL CANCER

The second most common skin cancer, squamous cell, also arises from the epidermis. They can occur on all areas of the body, including mucous membrane, but most commonly on sun-exposed areas. Detected and treated early, squamous cell cancer is highly curable. It is, however, more aggressive and more serious than basal cell cancer because it is more likely to invade structures beneath the skin. Squamous cell cancers sometimes follow a precancerous condition, called solar keratosis—rough patches that develop on heavily sun-exposed areas.

MALIGNANT MELANOMA

The incidence of melanoma, the most serious type of skin cancer, is increasing steadily. There has, in fact, been a 100 percent increase in melanoma since 1980, making it the fastest-increasing cancer around the world. Interestingly, the incidence is increasing fastest in women under the age of forty and the death rate for men over fifty is increasing faster than any other U.S. cancer. Although melanoma accounts for just 5 percent of skin cancer cases, it is responsible for 75 percent of deaths due to skin cancer.

Melanomas are cancers of the melanocytes (pigment-forming cells). They can occur on any part of the body where melanocytes exist, including the eye, nasal cavity, and vagina, but are most common on the skin.

There are four main clinical variants of malignant melanoma of the skin:

1. Lentigo Maligna Melanoma: This type of melanoma is characteristically found on the face, most commonly in elderly patients who have spent much time in the sun. Frequently there has been a dark, slowly growing area on the cheek, sometimes for as long as twenty years.

2. Superficial Spreading Melanoma: This is the most common type of melanoma in both the United States and Europe, typically striking people in the fourth and fifth decades of life. In the initial growth phase, this

tumor may resemble a simple mole, usually occurring on the leg in females and the trunk in males.

3. Nodular Melanoma: These are melanomas in which nodule formation is the first clinically visible sign of the cancer. Patients tend to be about the same age or younger than superficial-spreading melanoma patients. Nodular melanomas typically occur on areas of the body usually covered by clothing.

4. Acral Lentiginous Melanoma: The great majority of these cancers are found on the soles of the feet and the palms of the hands, usually in middle aged persons. This type of cancer is relatively rare among whites, accounting for 10 to 25 percent of melanomas, but is the most common type of melanoma among blacks and orientals. Acral lentiginous melanoma is believed to be unrelated to sun exposure.

There are two major risk factors for melanoma, pigmentation and sun exposure. Sun exposure, in fact, is believed to be the major environmental risk factor for melanoma of the skin in whites. It is generally assumed that the ultraviolet radiation associated with sunlight is the important factor, because ultraviolet radiation can cause cancer in experimental animals and in humans, and because melanin (the pigment in melanocytes) absorbs ultraviolet light.

The following evidence is important in suggesting the role of sun exposure.

1. Increased rates of melanoma in more southern locations, where ultraviolet light exposure is greater.

2. Increased risk among fair-skinned persons.

3. Low rates on sites unexposed to the sun.

4. Increased rates of occurrence, which could be due to changes in leisure sun exposure and in the social desirability of appearing tanned.

5. Sex/site-specific increases apparently reflecting changes in dress and resultant sun exposure.

Current evidence suggests that sun exposure can cause melanoma in two ways. Cumulative exposure to the sun, over a period of years, increases the risk of lentigo maligna melanoma and superficial and nodular melanomas of the head and neck. Intense, occasional exposure of untanned skin increases the risk of superficial spreading and nodular melanoma of other sites. As mentioned above, acral lentiginous melanoma does not appear to be related to sun exposure.

Instant Sunlight

The latest craze to hit the country is the tanning booth—an expensive form of solar outhouse, the only difference being that in this case, the hole is in the customer's head, not in the seat. Imported from Europe to accommodate those who just can't wait for summer, tanning booths provide a brief but intensive dose of ultraviolet radiation for an "all-over" tan.

Unfortunately, this type of radiation exposure is possibly the worst in terms of adverse health effects. Face and hands can quickly take on the appealing look of aged parchment with repeated visits. Eyes are also very vulnerable to this high-intensity radiation, even with goggles, as they don't offer 100 percent protection. Also, normally covered parts of the body are frequently exposed in the privacy of the tanning booth, and they are particularly susceptible to burning. Backing into a hot bulb is no fun, either.

Perhaps worst of all, this kind of ultraviolet exposure increases the risk of skin cancers more than does natural sunlight, since tanning booths don't come with a handy ozone layer for protection.

How to Reduce Your Risk of Skin Cancer

1. Don't broil yourself in the sun. This is especially important for fair-skinned people, but the common sense approach applies to everyone.

2. If you are going to sit in direct summer sunlight for more than fifteen minutes, use sunscreen or cover up. Fair-skinned people should use sunscreens during outdoor activities that expose areas of skin usually covered by clothing. Choose a sunscreen based on sunburn and tanning history. All sunscreen preparations are rated according to the amount of protection (Sun Protection Factor, SPF) they provide. Table 5.1 shows the recommended SPF for each type of skin. Remember to reapply sunscreen after swimming, heavy sweating, or if you will be out for more than a couple of hours. In addition to using sunscreens, people whose skins are sensitive to sun should wear protective clothing and/or avoid the sun during the summer between the hours of 10 A.M. and 3 P.M. when the ultraviolet rays are strongest.

Table 5.1
Skin Types and
Recommended Sunscreen Protection Factor

Skin type	Sensitivity to UV*	Sunburn and Tanning History	Recommended Sun Protection Factor**
I	Extremely sensitive	Always burns, never tans	15–30 or more
II	Very sensitive	Burns easily; tans minimally	15–30 or more
III	Sensitive	Burns moderately; tans gradually to a light brown	8–15
IV	Minimally sensitive	Burns minimally; always tans well to a dark brown	8–15
V	Not sensitive	Never burns	8–15

*Based on first 30 to 45 minutes' sun exposure after winter season or no sun exposure.
**Lower values for casual exposure and higher values for prolonged exposure.
Source: American Academy of Dermatology, 1990.

3. Do not use baby oil or mineral oil in the sun. They offer no protection and actually accelerate the burning process.

4. Start out sunbathing for a fifteen-minute period (with the sun screen), and increase your exposure gradually—five minutes each day—always with sunscreen.

5. Look out for cloudy days, too. Ultraviolet rays can penetrate almost anything. The "scatter" caused by moisture droplets in the air can allow 80 percent or more of the ultraviolet radiation to come through.

6. Remember that beach umbrellas only block out 50 to 55 percent of the sun's rays. You are exposed to

the rest of them from reflections off the sand and water.

7. Be especially cautious of sunlight in tropical countries and at high altitudes. Higher elevation means a thinner protective ozone layer—every thousand feet above sea level means you are exposed to 5 percent more ultraviolet rays.

8. Watch out for the sun when you ski—snow reflects about 80 percent of the sun's ultraviolet rays.

9. Don't use reflectors or oils to accelerate tanning.

10. Bring some light-colored clothing along with you when you go to the beach. If you burn easily, bring along a hat, too.

11. Lifeguards and others who spend long periods of time in the sun should consider using total-blocking agents such as zinc oxide and titanium dioxide.

Secondary Prevention

The second line of defense is to be aware of changes in one's skin. A five-minute monthly self-examination of the entire body using both a full length mirror and a hand-held mirror should be adequate to detect important skin changes. (See table 5.2 below.) A blow dryer on a cool setting can be used to expose the scalp. Medical attention should be sought if a new "mole" appears in adulthood or if changes are noted in an existing mole. Moles that are asymmetrical (cannot be divided into identical halves with an imaginary line), have uneven borders, are multi-colored, or are wider than a pencil eraser, should be brought to the attention of a dermatologist or other physician with expertise in skin disorders. If malignant melanoma is detected early enough, the rate of cure is excellent.

Table 5.2
Signs and Symptoms of Skin Cancers

Basal Cell Cancers

First appear as small round or oval patches, shiny and firm, usually white or gray, but sometimes pink or red.

Squamous Cell Cancers

Can be quite variable in their appearance, but are usually small, round, slightly raised, and red and crusty. Often there is a sore in the center that does not heal.

Melanomas

Although they can occur anywhere on the skin, they often occur where there is a mole. Be especially vigilant to any changes in your moles. According to the American Cancer Society, the ABCD rule can be used to help tell a normal mole or other marking from one that could be a melanoma. **ABCD** stands for:

Asymmetry—One half does not match the other.

Border Irregularity—The edges of the mole are ragged, notched, or blurred.

Color—The color is not the same over all of the mole, but may be differing shades of tan, brown, or black, sometimes with patches of red, white, or blue.

Diameter—The mole is wider than 6 millimeters (¼") or is growing larger.

6

Radiation
Managing Technology Safely

During the early 1900s young women employed in watch manufacturing factories painted luminous dials on watch faces using a material containing radium. In the course of their work these women commonly "tipped" the end of their brushes using their tongue and lips. This resulted in ingestion of significant amounts of radiation. Of some seventeen hundred workers employed in this trade, forty-eight died from bone cancer. Normally, less than one person would be expected to die from bone cancer in a population more than twice that size.

Unfortunately, watch-dial painters were not the only unsuspecting victims of excessive radiation in the days before its hazard was known. About fifteen thousand British patients treated with high levels of radiation in hopes of alleviating the great discomfort of ankylosing spondylitis (a painful disease that causes the spine to stiffen) were administered doses of x-rays averaging 370,000 millirads. This procedure resulted in ten times more leukemia deaths than would normally be expected. (Whelan 1978)

The atomic-bomb attack on Japan that ended World War II not only killed many people, but also, sadly, presented the medical community with unique long-term health problems. Thousands of survivors had been exposed to doses of radiation much greater than normal background levels. Medical and epidemiologic follow-up has enabled us to learn a great deal about radiation's effects on human health and on the levels of radiation necessary to cause those effects.

Radiation is now a proven cause of human cancer. But, as with all of the other carcinogens discussed in this book, it's the dose that makes the poison. While excessive doses do cause human cancer, there is no evidence that the normally small amounts that occur naturally or that are emitted from various man-made technologies are increasing the cancer burden.

Let's look at the doses we're exposed to, and also at the amounts known to cause cancer.

Measuring Human Radiation Exposure: Terminology

Radiation terminology is difficult to understand, but essential in any discussion of radiation exposure. Here are the basics:

rad: amount of radiation absorbed per gram of body tissue.

gray: 100 rad (an international term for rad, gradually replacing the rad).

rem: a term that expresses the damage potential of any particular type of radiation dose; the rad is multiplied by a quality factor to determine the rem.

sievert: international unit expressing damage potential of any particular type of radiation dose.

How Much Radiation Are We Exposed To?

On the average, Americans annually are exposed to approximately one-third rem, or 360 millirems of radiation from all sources, including naturally occurring radiation, medical uses, radiation from consumer products, radiation from occupational activities, nuclear power production, and miscellaneous environmental sources (including fallout from nuclear weapons testing).

By far the largest contributor to this dose is natural background radiation, contributing 82 percent. It has recently been estimated that as much as two-thirds of this natural background dose is caused by radon and its decay products. The other third is equally divided among cosmic radiation, terrestrial radiation, and internally deposited radionuclides.

Medical procedures contribute approximately 18 percent of the annual dose (smaller than previously estimated) and consumer products about 3 percent.

Radiation from occupational activities, the entire nuclear power process, and other miscellaneous sources, including fallout from nuclear weapons testing, *together* account for less than one percent of our annual exposure, or less than one one-thousandth of a rem.

Natural Radiation

Radiation exists naturally in the environment. The amount present in a specific place is primarily determined by the geography and topography of the region. Cosmic rays that originate from the sun are one of the two major sources of natural radiation. Solar cosmic rays are protons accelerated by electric and magnetic fields around the sun. The atmosphere serves as an absorber for most of the sun's cosmic rays. Therefore, the amount of radiation exposure from the sun increases in proportion to altitude.

Radioactive material within the earth's crust is the other major source of natural radiation. A number of elements including potassium, radium, uranium, and thorium contain isotopes that are naturally radioactive. The average layer of soil measuring one foot deep and one mile square (1.7 million tons of soil) contains four to five tons of uranium, six tons of thorium, and one gram of radium. Some of the decay products of these elements are gases that continually escape from the soil. Most radiation comes directly from the ground, from building materials, and from radioactive materials inside our bodies, such as radioactive potassium in muscles. (Cobb 1989)

Because of these factors, the overall background radiation doses in cities or regions differ greatly. For example, Denver has almost twice the natural background radiation than is found in most spots in Florida.

Some inhabited areas of Brazil have measured levels of background radiation six times the average for the United States. In fact, plants growing on a hill in the state of Minas Gerais absorb so much radioactive material from the soil that they can be x-rayed simply by placing their leaves in contact with x-ray film.

Radiation and Adverse Health Effects*

As with all toxic substances, the degree of hazard of radiation is dependent upon the dose or exposure. Radiation is dangerous in high doses. At very high doses, about four thousand times annual background-radiation dose, radiation can cause acute sickness and death. At doses which are lower, but above one hundred times the annual background dose, an increased risk of cancer has been observed.

Information about the types of disease caused by excessive radiation exposure and the doses of radiation necessary to induce acute illness and cancer has been gathered by studying a number of occupationally exposed groups, patients subject to inappropriate therapeutic use, and survivors of the atomic bombs dropped on Japan during World War II.

By comparing the intensity of radiation exposure in a given area with the resulting numbers of fatalities, researchers found that a single exposure to 1 million millirads will be lethal to everyone, and a 450,000-millirad exposure will cause about half of the exposed population to die within a month. (Eisenbud 1978)

Cancer and reproduction patterns among a hundred thousand survivors of the atomic attack on Nagasaki were studied by the Radiation Effects Research Foundation (RERF). (Sagan 1979) Average exposure had been 20,000 millirads per person, or the equivalent of four hundred chest x-rays. RERF found that the increase in cancer incidence caused by the radiation exposure at this level was minimal, the

---

*See also the section on radiation and the nuclear power industry in chapter 11.

radiation accounting for just one of every five hundred cases of cancer in the exposed group.

Human reproduction was also affected by the radiation shower in Japan. Women pregnant at the time of exposure gave birth to a higher than expected percentage of children with birth defects. An increased incidence of genetic defects has been seen in offspring of animals exposed to radiation in laboratory studies. However, such genetic effects have not been shown for the Japanese A-bomb survivors. According to a *National Geographic* in-depth review:

> Surprisingly no genetic evidence suggests generations to come are doomed. Tests on mice and fruit flies show harmful results. So why not humans? Spontaneous abortions, perhaps, or some remedial effect of the lengthy human gestation period. Said Dr. [Jacob] Thiessen [of RERF], "We would like to find some directly measurable effect. Right now we don't see anything." (Cobb 1989)

Scientists now know that excess radiation will causes certain types of cancers—in particular leukemia, lung, breast, and stomach cancer (but generally not pancreatic, prostate, cervical, or uterine cancer)—some twenty to thirty years after the exposure.

Radiation Levels That Will Cause Cancer

As a result of epidemiologic studies done on human populations after the above-mentioned episodes, we know that radiation at relatively high doses can cause cancer, birth defects, and other adverse health effects. The key issue, then, is whether people in the general environment are exposed to hazardous levels. Fortunately, those exposed to environmental background radiation have experienced few health problems from this background radiation. For example, residents of Denver receive twice the U.S. average (because of their high altitude), yet they have one of the lowest overall cancer rates in the United States.

A cause-and-effect relationship between radiation and cancer has been shown only at levels above 20,000 millirads, with the most solid evidence from exposure of 100,000 millirads or more. As the level of radiation exposure decreases, the evidence of a carcinogenic effect becomes less detectable. Most studies on the human health effects of lower levels of radiation reach the same conclusion—there is no convincing evidence that a single exposure to 20,000 millirads or less will cause cancer. There have been some studies, in fact, which show a beneficial effect of low-level radiation. However, to be on the safe side, regulations regarding radiation doses are based on the assumption that the effects of radiation are proportional to the dose even at levels below which no effects have been observed.

Radiation from Medical Procedures

Some people have tried to estimate the amount of cancer due to x-rays and other medical procedures that utilize radiation. But, according to Fred Mettler, M.D., Chief of Radiology at the University of New Mexico and U.S. Representative to the United Nations Scientific Committee on the Effects of Radiation, it may be nearly impossible to estimate this contribution. The United Nations and other international groups have been unwilling to come up with an estimate.

Some figures you might see indicate that medical pro-cedures are responsible for one-half of one percent of all cancer cases in this country. This, says Dr. Mettler, is most likely a gross overestimate. The actual percentage could be zero, or it could be somewhere between 0 and 0.5 percent.

Common sense dictates that while we wouldn't want to avoid a medical procedure (such as one that utilizes radiation) if we need it, we also don't want to undergo any unnecessary medical tests, especially those involving radiation. Prudent use of medical diagnostic procedures will not only save precious health care dollars, but may in the final analysis prevent unnecessary exposure to radiation.

To Reduce Your Risks of Cancer

1. If the best medical advice indicates you should have a test involving radiation, you should, of course, have that test. Do ask that the technician place appropriate protective shields over vulnerable areas of the body, such as over the reproductive organs.

2. Avoid unnecessary radiologic tests, and don't insist on tests that your doctor deems unnecessary.

7

Sexual and Reproductive Patterns

Isn't there any pleasurable aspect of life that doesn't increase the risk of cancer? Does sex cause cancer, too?

Evidence gathered over the past four hundred years clearly suggests that certain patterns of sexual and reproductive behavior can increase your likelihood of cancers of the breast, cervix, and uterus. Less markedly, sexual behavior may also affect the risks for cancers of the penis and prostate gland. Recently, it has also been determined that sexual activity can increase the risk of Acquired Immune Deficiency Syndrome (AIDS).

Some of the associations noted between sexual and reproductive behavior and cancer incidence have little practical application because they are based on biological aspects of our lives over which we have little control. Others do have limited application—if not for you in particular, then perhaps for the next generations of your family.

You might argue that sexual and reproductive patterns are not "environmental" in origin. But these lifestyle factors are more a product of choice than of genetics.

Breast Cancer

Breast cancer is the second most common cancer in American women. According to American Cancer Society estimates, over 180,000 cases of breast cancer were diagnosed in the United States in 1993. About one out of eight women will develop breast cancer during their lives, and one out of twenty-eight will die from it. There are a number of known risk factors for breast cancer that relate to sexual and reproductive patterns.

Unmarried women, for example, are at increased risk of breast cancer. This observation was one of the first epidemiological correlations ever made. In the 1700s, cloistered nuns were noted to have elevated rates of breast cancer. Indeed, one researcher in 1842 wrote "that cancers are more frequent in nuns than other women at a ratio of about five to one." In fact, this is true for all unmarried women. But the explanation for this is not the fact that they are leading "celibate lives," but rather because they have not had any children.

Not only does it make a difference whether or not you've had a child, but your age at the birth of your first child has a part in determining your risk. The longer a woman waits to have her first child, the more likely she is to develop breast cancer later in life. In the 1990s, we also know that earlier age at the birth of a second child further reduces the risk of breast cancer.

Women who have their first child after the age of thirty have a twofold increase of breast cancer compared to women whose first child was born before the age of twenty. More recent evidence, however, points to a complex pattern regarding age at first birth: there is a transiently increased risk relative to that for a woman who has never given birth that lasts for one to two decades, followed by a lower risk later in life. (When you compare that to the four- to tenfold increase in lung cancer risk associated with cigarette smoking, you can see that this association is much less important in terms of cancer prevention).

There are other risk factors for breast cancer that are outside of our own individual control and have nothing to do with sexual and reproductive patterns. For example, age is a critical factor: the rate of breast cancer is a leading cause of death among American women forty to fifty years of age. The risk of breast cancer is increased among women who have a family history of the disease. A woman's risk is increased approximately twofold if her mother or sister have it and four- to sixfold if two first-degree relatives have it, such as a mother and sister or two sisters. This risk grows if the first-degree relative has cancer in both breasts, and also if the cancer occurs before the age of fifty.

There has been some controversy about the effect of fibrocystic disease on a woman's future risk of breast cancer. Until the mid 1980s, it was thought that a woman with fibrocystic breasts had a three- to fivefold increase in breast cancer. In the 1990s, however, doctors believe that women whose benign breast lumps show no abnormalities (medically speaking, no proliferative changes) have little or no increased risk. Generally speaking, just 4 to 10 percent of women with benign breast lumps have, on microscopic exam, those proliferative changes that may increase breast cancer risk.

BREAST FEEDING

There is conflicting evidence about the protective effect of breast feeding.

Since early in this century there has been speculation that nursing may be related to lower breast cancer risk. As one physician wrote in 1926, "The breast which has never been called upon for normal function is certainly more liable to become cancerous." The evidence of risk reduction, however, becomes questionable because it is confused with the effect of having a child (which is a proven protection). If breast feeding does offer immunity, the strongest evidence in the 1990s is for premenopausal breast cancer cases. But, again, research results on this issue have not yet met on common ground.

WEIGHING THE RISKS OF BREAST CANCER*

The fact that age of first birth affects a woman's likelihood of getting breast cancer is of little practical use. If a woman believes in the traditional means of starting a family and doesn't get married until later in life, she doesn't have the opportunity to have children at an early age.

Other information we have about risk factors for breast cancer have even less practical application. For example, women who begin menstruating early in life, that is before age twelve, have a higher risk of breast cancer than those who mature later. This may be due to nutritional factors, since improved nutritional status is believed to be associated with early onset of the menses. Women who reach menopause

---

*See also chapter 8 on estrogen and cancer risk.

later than age fifty-five also have a doubled risk compared to women who reach natural menopause before age forty-five. Presumably this is because these women are exposed to the hormone stimulus that may be causing the disease for longer periods of time. Women who have their ovaries removed before age forty have lowered risk of breast cancer—surgical menopause is associated with a 40 percent reduction in risk.

These observations don't do much to help you in avoiding cancer, but they are useful to scientists in the development of new hypotheses. If we better understood the hormonal aspects of breast cancer, perhaps women could be offered some preventive measures.

The role of women in society has changed dramatically in the past decade due to the political and economic dynamics of society. But as many women are learning, there are often unforeseen costs associated with these changes. One such cost may be incurred by delaying childbearing well into the third or even fourth decade of life. Given the current trend among American women to delay childbearing in favor of career pursuits, will breast cancer mortality among premenopausal women begin to rise toward the end of the century? Should a young woman choose to minimize her long-term health risk by bearing a child at a relatively young age, or should she instead minimize her long-term economic risk by settling into a career? If these questions are indeed relevant, one suspects they are unanswerable. One also suspects, however, that given the option, most women would rather confront the dilemma than return to the simpler and more repressive good old days.

CERVICAL CANCER

The cervix is the small cylindrical neck that leads from the uterus, or womb, into the vagina. A portion of the cervix protrudes into the vagina and can be easily seen during a gynecological examination. A sample of cells can be taken for examination (The Pap test) and cellular changes sometimes associated with cancer detected. Some 13,500 cases of cervical cancer were diagnosed in 1993, with 4,400 associated deaths. Although the incidence of invasive cervical cancer has decreased by almost 50 percent since 1945, the incidence of precancerous lesions has increased dramatically, and is occurring in younger and younger women and girls. It is estimated that 1.8 to 2.8 percent of women aged fifteen to nineteen have precancerous cervical lesions.

In 1993, there is no question that high-risk sexual behavior—that is, having more than one sexual partner—is the most important cause of cervical cancer. It has become increasingly clear that cervical cancer is caused, in whole or in part, by one or more sexually transmitted agents, most likely the human papillomaviruses (HPVs). Early evidence, somewhat unexplained at the time, now makes sense: prostitutes studied while in prison in the 1960s were found to have a four- to sevenfold increase in cervical cancer over other female inmates. Other early evidence came from Dr. Irving Kessler, a Johns Hopkins professor of epidemiology, who noted that women married to widowers whose previous wives died from cervical cancer had four times the frequency of this disease as compared to a closely matched group of women.

HUMAN PAPILLOMAVIRUSES

Human papillomaviruses (HPVs) are a group of more than seventy types of viruses. They are called papillomaviruses because they tend to cause warts, or papillomas, that are benign (noncancerous) tumors. Different types of HPVs cause the common warts that grow on hands and feet and those that develop in the mouth and genital area.

Some genital HPVs can be passed from one person to another through sexual intercourse and oral or anal sex. Nonsexual routes of transmission are also possible. Genital HPVs may cause warts to appear on or around the genitals and anus of both men and women. In women, they may also appear in the cervix. This type of a "genital wart" is known technically as condyloma acuminatum.

Some HPVs, such as HPV-6 and HPV-11, are often referred to as "low risk" viruses, as they develop into cancer relatively less frequently. Other sexually transmitted HPVs that have been linked with cancers in both men and women are referred to as "high-risk"; they include HPV-16 and HPV-18 and have been found in the anus and on the genitals (including the vulva and penis).

Both high-risk and low-risk types of HPVs can cause the growth of abnormal cells in the cervix. Abnormal cells can be detected when the doctor does a Pap smear during a regular gynecologic exam. Several different terms have been used to describe the abnormal cells that may be seen in Pap smears. In the Bethesda system (one system used to report the results of Pap smears), precancerous conditions are called low-grade and high-grade squamous intraepithelial lesions. Squamous cells are thin, flat cells resembling fish scales that are found in the tissue that forms the surface of the skin, the lining of the hollow organs of the body such as the cervix, and the passages of the respiratory and digestive tracts. Other terms sometimes used to describe these abnormal cells are cervical intraepithelial neoplasia and dysplasia. Low-grade, or minor, dysplasia is a fairly common condition, especially in young women.

There is currently no cure for a papillomavirus infection. Only the symptoms can be treated. The warts and abnormal cell growth these viruses cause can be removed with cold cautery (freezing that destroys tissue), hot cautery (burning warts off with an electrical instrument), and laser treatment (surgery with a high-intensity light), as well as conventional surgery. In addition, two powerful chemicals (podophyllin and trichloracetic acid) will destroy genital warts when applied directly to them.

Not removed, these cells will cause cancer in some women. Studies suggest that whether a person will develop cancer depends on a variety of factors that act together with HPVs. These factors include smoking, decreased resistance to infection, and infection with agents other than HPVs. In addition, behaviors that increase a person's chance of getting an HPV infection, such as beginning sexual intercourse at an early age and having many sexual partners, are risk factors for the development of cervical cancer.

HERPES VIRUS 2

Over the past twenty years, there has been increasing evidence that the herpes virus type 2 (HSV-2) may be a causative agent in cervical cancer.

Herpes viruses are more commonly known for causing cold sores, or fever blisters, in the mouth region (type 1 herpes virus), and for causing venereal lesions (herpes virus type 2).

Herpes virus type 2, which strikes in the genital region, is now occurring with increasing frequency in both sexes. Not only is it occurring in epidemic proportions, it is also incurable.

Herpes lesions occur on or near the sex organs some three days after sex with an infected person. The sores take the form of clusters of small blisters which can break in a day or two, to form shallow ulcers. The disease usually clears up without treatment, within about six weeks, and leaves no scar. But during the course of the disease the patient may feel burning and pain, fever, or a "flu-like" illness. Repeat attacks of herpes frequently occur over the next few years without new venereal contact; the disease is chronic and recurrent. Attacks may be precipitated by anything—emotional or physical trauma, menstruation, or other illness. The second attack is usually less severe and shorter in duration than the first. There is no specific treatment, but bathing with a weak salt solution may relieve discomfort. As with any venereal disease, the primary means of prevention is avoidance of contact with an affected person.

Studies of women in several geographical areas have provided evidence that antibodies to HSV-2, which are indicative of previous or current infection, occur significantly more frequently in women with cancer of the cervix than in those free of the disease. Prospective studies, which have followed large numbers of women over a period of years have found that women who initially have genital herpes or antibody to HSV-2 are more likely to develop cervical cancer or tissue abnormalities than are women who have not been infected with HSV-2. Samples of cells taken from cervical cancer patients have also shown evidence of the presence of HSV-2, further implicating the virus as a culprit. Related herpes viruses have been shown to cause tumors in animals, and it is thought that Burkitt's lymphoma, a cancer found in African children, is caused by human herpes virus. Thus, it is logical that among women who have early and frequent intercourse with a number of different men, the herpes virus may initiate or promote cancer of the cervix.

In a sexually free society where attitudes and behavior have changed dramatically over the past decades, the question of an association between cancer of the cervix and herpes 2 obviously merits further investigation. Not only are young women having sex earlier, but the oral contraceptive is widely used instead of barrier forms of contraception; only the latter might offer some protection when properly used.

Uterus

Some of the risk factors for uterine cancer, also called endometrial cancer, are the same as those for breast cancer. For example, many of the risk factors may be related to hormonal imbalances. Infertility, particularly characterized by the lack of ovulation, and obesity are particularly distinctive risk factors for this type of cancer. Women developing endometrial cancer at a relatively young age often have a medical history of menstrual irregularities and infertility. Age at menopause in endometrial patients is on the average later than that observed among other women.

Sexually Related Cancer in Males

Cancer of the penis is very rare in the United States. It occurs most frequently in areas of the world where circumcision is not routinely practiced, and where penile hygiene is poor. We have little information regarding what causes this type of cancer.

Prostate cancer is a leading cause of male cancer death in this country. Diet, and the resulting stimulation of the gland by hormones, probably plays a more important role in prostate cancer causation than does sexual behavior. The few epidemiological studies that have been done on prostate cancer suggest that sexual factors might play a small role, though. Married men have a somewhat higher rate of this disease than do single men.

AIDS

AIDS, or Acquired Immune Deficiency Syndrome, cripples an important part of the body's immune system. This leaves a person vulnerable to infections (often rare and/or of a mild nature in noninfected people) and also to cancer.

The most common "opportunistic" infection contracted by AIDS victims is a severe type of pneumonia caused by the parasite *pneumocystis carinii*. *Pneumocystis carinii* pneumonia (PCP) very rarely occurs among individuals with normally functioning immune systems.

Persons with AIDS are also likely to develop other serious infections caused by bacteria, fungi, viruses, and parasites. Infection by such organisms may be responsible for the development of pneumonia, meningitis, encephalitis, esophagitis, persistent diarrhea and extensive skin inflammation among AIDS victims. PCP and these other opportunistic infections are often resistant to treatment and are frequently the immediate cause of death of AIDS victims.

AIDS and Cancer

Over a decade into the AIDS crisis, we now know that AIDS patients are particularly prone to developing certain types of cancer, including some ordinarily very rare in occurrence. Some of these cancers are Kaposi's sarcoma, non-Hodgkin's lymphoma, and primary lymphoma of the brain.

KAPOSI'S SARCOMA

Until the AIDS epidemic, Kaposi's sarcoma (KS) was a rare tumor affecting predominantly elderly males of eastern European or Mediterranean Jewish descent. KS was one of the first disorders recognized to occur with AIDS, and was, at one point, the second most common illness in AIDS patients. In the 1990s, other AIDS complications, including *pneumocystis carinii* and yeast infections, have become more common than KS. Nevertheless, the number of KS cases continues to grow, and KS will continue to be a major reason for serious illness and death among AIDS patients.

KS is a cancer originating in the body's blood vessels, and appearing as dark blue or purple-brown plaques (spots) or bumps, most commonly on the lower extremities. They can, however, occur anywhere on the skin or mucous membranes. This cancer spreads quickly. Approximately 30 percent of patients with AIDS are first diagnosed when they go to the doctor with these skin lesions, and, in fact, the diagnosis of KS in an otherwise healthy person continues to be a major CDC criterion for the diagnosis of AIDS.

NON-HODGKIN'S LYMPHOMA

AIDS patients have a twenty-five- to one-hundred-fold increase in Non-Hodgkin's lymphoma (NHL) over the general population; in addition, NHL among them is very aggressive and usually has a poorer prognosis that when it affects non-AIDS patients. As is typical of AIDS, the rarer sub-types of NHL are more common among AIDS patients than among non-AIDS patients; similarly, this cancer may infect unusual sites as well. It has been estimated that by the mid 1990s, AIDS patients will make up nearly 80 percent of all people with NHL.

One of the theories about NHL among AIDS patients is that they are more seriously affected by the Epstein-Barr virus, which, somehow, leads to NHL. The Epstein-Barr virus is found in 20 to 70 percent of HIV-related lymphomas.

PRIMARY LYMPHOMA OF THE BRAIN

Approximately 3 percent of AIDS patients will develop primary lymphoma of the brain, which will be diagnosed before they die. An additional 3 percent are found to have this type of cancer only when an autopsy is conducted (in other words, it went undiagnosed prior to their death). The vast majority of these cases comprise what is known as an AIDS-defining illness, i.e., an illness with which AIDS is diagnosed.

AIDS represents the single most common reason why an increase in this type of cancer has been noted over the past several years. Since 1982, in fact, its occurrence has more than tripled in the United States and Great Britain. In some United States centers, there has even been a six- to fifteenfold increase between 1983 and 1990 compared to the prior twenty years.

The symptoms include headaches, numbness in the face, seizures, partial paralysis, and personality change. Some patients may go to the doctor simply because they have a change in their personality, such as suddenly becoming inexplicably apathetic.

CERVICAL CANCER

There is some evidence that AIDS infected women have a higher incidence of cervical cancer. One theory is that the HIV infection somehow interacts with the human papillomavirus (HPV) infection to increase the chance of developing cervical cancer even over that of women who are infected with HPV.

ANAL CANCER

There have been some reports of increased risk of anal cancer among homosexual men who test positive for both HIV and HPV.

MALIGNANT LYMPHOMA OF THE HEART

Also an extremely rare cancer, malignant lymphomas of the heart are occurring with increasing frequency in AIDS patients. AIDS patients with this type of cancer generally develop serious heart symptoms, including heart failure and irregular heartbeat, which progress very quickly.

Hepatitis B and Liver Cancer

There is no questions that Hepatitis B (HBV) is a dangerous infectious agent and a threat to public health. In the United States alone, 200,000 to 300,000 new infections with this virus occur each year. Among other things, a high-risk lifestyle—relevant to this chapter is homosexual activity—significantly increases the chances of acquiring HBV.

HBV infection may result in a range of clinical courses. After a two- to six-month incubation period, HBV can lead to "acute hepatitis." (Hepatitis, of which there are 5 forms, is an inflammation of the liver.) If the body is unable to mount an effective immune response, a patient may become a chronic carrier of HBV. Chronic carriers are at increased risk of developing cirrhosis of the liver and hepatocellular carcinoma, a dangerous liver cancer. In fact, HBV is said by many scientists to be "second only to tobacco as a known human carcinogen."

How to Reduce Your Risk of Cancer

WOMEN: PRIMARY PREVENTION

1. Postpone intercourse until you choose one partner for life.

2. If practical, have your first child before you are thirty.

WOMEN: SECONDARY PREVENTION

1. Have a regular Pap test and pelvic exam.

MEN

1. Postpone intercourse until you choose one partner for life.

MEN AND WOMEN

1. If you are an IV drug user:

  - get professional help in kicking the drug habit.

  - if you are unable to get off drugs, do not share needles and syringes (boiling water does not guarantee sterility). You should also be aware that drug merchants may sell previously used needles as new.
  - avoid sexual contact (homosexual or heterosexual) with anyone who uses IV drugs or is in any other way at risk for AIDS.

2. Don't share toothbrushes, razors, or other implements that could become contaminated with blood from anyone who has, or might have, AIDS.

3. Avoid procedures, such as acupuncture or tattooing, in which needles and other unsterile instruments are used repeatedly for piercing skin and/or mucous membranes.

4. If you are a health care worker:

  - be extremely careful to avoid accidental wounds from sharp instruments contaminated with potentially infectious material and to avoid contact of open skin lesions with material from AIDS patients.

- wear gloves and other protective clothing if you might be exposed to an AIDS patient's blood, wastes, secretions, etc. Depending on the extent of your potential exposure, you may need a mask, eye covering, and gown, in addition to gloves.
- Wash your hands after removing protective clothing and before leaving the room of known or suspected AIDS patients. Wash your hands immediately if they become contaminated with the blood or other secretion of an AIDS patient.
- Be sure to label blood and other specimens from AIDS patients prominently with a special warning. Wash the outside of the container if it becomes contaminated. Place all specimens inside a second leak-proof container for transport.
- If you provide emergency medical care, check into the availability of "S-tubes" or hand resuscitator bags for use in administering artificial respiration.
- Follow all recommended procedures in your institution or office *exactly.*

8

Medicines

In the late 1940s, a couple I'll call Jim and Susan Peterson, and their five-year-old son, moved to the Boston suburbs. The Petersons had always wanted a large family—five children, at least. But things didn't work out as they had planned. Not until after ten years of marriage was their first child born. Before her son's birth, she had several miscarriages, and when he was born Susan was eager to seek another pregnancy as soon as possible.

In 1949, Susan became pregnant again, and this time her obstetrician decided to take no chances. He prescribed a new drug-diethylstilbestrol or stilbestrol as it was frequently called—which apparently worked wonders in cases where miscarriage had occurred several times. Given Susan's age, thirty-six, and history of pregnancy loss, he felt that stilbestrol was indicated. Immediately after her pregnancy was confirmed, she started on stilbestrol pills, and used them at particularly high doses during the first trimester.

Susan had a daughter, Anna, who was normal at birth

and enjoyed a happy childhood. In 1970, Anna graduated from high school and entered college that fall. In late September she began to experience heavy vaginal bleeding between menstrual periods, but didn't take it too seriously. Many girls had noticed menstrual changes that started when they entered college. The bleeding stopped for awhile, but then became progressively heavier through December. While home on Christmas vacation, she was examined by a gynecologist in Boston, who found some unusual vaginal ridges. And her cervix was an odd, bright red color. After a biopsy was taken, the results showed that Anna had a rare cancer of the vagina—adenocarcinoma. She underwent a full hysterectomy and vaginectomy (removal of the vagina).

DES—the "Miracle Drug"

In 1938, Dr. E. C. Dodds discovered a way of synthesizing a form of estrogen in the laboratory, which was greeted with great enthusiasm in the medical community. In the past, estrogens had only been available from pregnant mare's urine, or other natural sources. These were not only too expensive to prescribe for general use, but were also highly ineffective when taken orally.

The new, synthetic estrogen, stilbestrol, corrected these difficulties—it was easy to make, inexpensive, and could be taken in the form of a pill.

Stilbestrol seemed to hold the greatest promise in the area of treating menopausal symptoms. A November 1941 issue of *Today's Health* magazine praised the new drug, noting it was effective in relieving pain, discomfort, crying spells, sleeplessness, and "nerves." Medical journals raved that stilbestrol had "extraordinary clinical possibilities." In addition to being used as treatment for menopausal symptoms, stilbestrol was immediately seen as a drug to control prostate cancer.

Stilbestrol use steadily increased among older women and men with various symptoms of menopause and prostate cancer, and soon physicians had some expanded ideas for its use. In 1943, a doctor writing in *Medical Times* noted that while it was "outstanding" in managing menopausal symptoms, it should also be used in pregnancy testing, treatment of morning sickness, and treatment of threatened miscarriage.

By 1948, a whole series of medical journals were recommending the use of stilbestrol during pregnancy. Some writers in the late 1940s and 1950s went so far as to suggest that stilbestrol be given to all pregnant women, whether or not they had a history of miscarriage, to prevent or decrease the hazards of late complications of pregnancy for mothers and their babies. The stilbestrol therapy was particularly in favor at a prestigious medical center in Boston, and indeed it was there, some 20 years later that the first signs of a problem were noted.

Rumblings about the possible ineffectiveness of stilbestrol in pregnancy began in the early 1950s. Dr. R. Robinson and Dr. Landrum Shettles reported that "in careful comparisons . . . there was no evidence that stilbestrol increased the pregnancy salvage rate." In 1953, the evidence against stilbestrol became even stronger (although as yet, there was no mention of any harmful side effects of the drug). Gradually, use of the drug slowed, but as late as 1970, some obstetricians still prescribed the drug "to prevent miscarriage."

In 1966, Dr. Howard Ulfelder, a gynecologist at the

Vincent Memorial Hospital (part of the Massachusetts General Hospital), saw a sixteen-year-old girl with unusual vaginal bleeding patterns. He diagnosed adenocarcinoma of the vagina. This case was very puzzling to him, since cancer of the vagina is extremely rare, especially in women under the age of fifty. Between 1966 and 1970, seven girls, ages fifteen to twenty-two, were seen at the same hospital with the same disease.

Dr. Ulfelder and his associates confirmed that the victims did not all use any type of intravaginal irritant, douches, or tampons. Only one patient had had sexual intercourse, a known risk factor. None had used birth control pills before onset of the disease. By comparing the seven girls to other girls without the disease, they found a highly significant association between adenocarcinoma and the treatment of the victims' mothers during pregnancy with stilbestrol. All the mothers had begun taking stilbestrol in the first trimester of pregnancy.

The Boston doctors published their results in an April 1971 issue of the *New England Journal of Medicine*. This report came out thirty years after stilbestrol was first used as a drug in the United States, and twenty-eight years after the first suggestion that it be used in pregnancy.

It was the timing of the drug's use that was most critical to the future development of cancer. In the first three months of pregnancy, the fetal vaginal cells seem to be very sensitive to hormones, and may undergo the first malignant transformation.

How Many People Are at Risk?

It is believed that between four and six million Americans—mothers, daughters and sons—may have had pregnancy-related exposures to DES. (DES-using mothers themselves also had a slightly increased risk of breast cancer, but this effect is disappearing as we move further away from DES use.) Since early 1970 a few hundred cases of adenocarcinoma of the vagina have been reported to a central registry. There is no doubt now that there is a clear link between exposure to DES before birth and an increased risk of this type of cancer. But the good news is that the risk is nowhere near as high as originally feared. It is now estimated that no more than 1.4 per 1,000 exposed daughters up to the age of 24 will develop clear cell adenocarcinoma of the vagina or cervix. The rate may actually be as low as 1.4 per 10,000. There does not appear to be additional risk of developing any other types of cancer. One recent study found only four other cases of cancer among a total of more than 3,000 DES daughters examined.

In addition to being associated with a small number of cancers in the daughters of mothers using DES, anatomic abnormalities of the sperm and reproductive tract have been reported in sons. To date studies have not revealed whether or not these types of abnormalities have led to infertility problems in these males.

Postmenopausal Estrogen Therapy

Estrogens have been used in the treatment of menopausal symptoms for more than fifty years. Estrogen therapy is very effective in reducing those symptoms of menopause that are related to the decreasing body levels of estrogen. Taking estrogens for a short time while the body adjusts to its new hormone level frequently helps women with severe hot flashes or vaginal problems. Estrogens do not "cure" menopause; they simply help some women who have disabling symptoms get through it more easily. Women whose ovaries have been removed surgically early in their reproductive lives seem to suffer more severe hot flashes than do women who experience a natural menopause, and these women are especially good candidates for estrogen therapy. More importantly, estrogen helps prevent osteoporosis ("brittle bones") and heart disease.

Estrogen therapy has been proven helpful in slowing one aspect of the aging process. As bones age, they become less dense and more brittle. This condition, known as osteoporosis, makes bones more fragile and more prone to fractures. Bone fractures are a very significant health problem in elderly women. Twenty-five percent of white women older than sixty years develop spontaneous fractures of the vertebrae. One in six women who suffers a hip fracture at age ninety or above will die within three months of her injury.

One-fourth of all postmenopausal women in the United States develop an unhealthy degree of bone loss. It is difficult to predict, however, which women will experience these bone changes. Women who are chronically disabled or bedridden may indeed have bone loss problems that could be helped by estrogen therapy. On the other hand, black women and tall, diabetic or obese women usually do not suffer from osteoporosis.

Danish investigators reported in *Lancet* in 1981 that as little as two years of postmenopausal estrogen therapy resulted in prevention of bone loss. A 1982 study, reported in *Annals of Internal Medicine,* suggested that moderate doses of estrogen given over a two-year period prevent significant bone mineral loss in premenopausal women whose ovaries have been removed.

It must be emphasized that many other factors, in addition to estrogen, are important for healthy bones in postmenopausal women. Several other hormones, vitamin D, and calcium are all involved in the maintenance of normal bones. Genetics, body weight, exercise, diet and cigarette smoking are also factors that influence bone thickness.

Oral Contraceptives

There has been some research suggesting that oral contraceptives may cause breast cancer, although the results are not consistent. The best evidence indicates that if they do influence cancer development, they probably don't initiate cancer changes, but only accelerate those already there. Some evidence even points to oral contraceptives as retarding cells that have cancerous changes. Finally, some experts think there is some sub-group of the population that may be sensitive to the cancer-influencing ability of oral contraceptives.

Interestingly, there is extensive evidence pointing to the fact that oral contraceptives significantly reduce one's chances of developing endometrial cancer. According to the Centers for Disease Control and Prevention (CDC), oral contraceptives probably slash the risk of endometrial cancer in half, preventing some 2,000 cases per year. Women who have had no or few children apparently benefit the most, as they have the highest risk of endometrial cancer.

Cancer and Immunosuppressive Drugs

CANCER DRUGS

We all benefit enormously from the many life-saving cancer drugs now available. These "antineoplastic drugs," sometimes used in combination with radiation therapy and/or surgery, significantly prolong life and even yield remarkable cures for many cancer patients.

One of the most important points I hope to make in this book is that sometimes we have to accept some level of risk to benefit from something. In this case, some people have to accept the risk of developing a cancer distinct from their original disease as a result of taking cancer drugs.

The largest category of cancer-fighting drugs that may cause cancer at other sites are called alkylating agents, used for many types of cancers, including non-Hodgkin's lymphoma, malignant lymphomas, multiple myeloma, polycythemia, and solid tumors at various sties. Some of these agents are listed here:

- cyclophosphamide
- chorambucil
- busulfan
- dihydroxy-busulfan
- thiotepa
- treosulfan

Another category of cancer-fighting drugs, called nitrosureas may also be associated with leukemia, but not as strongly as the alkylating agents. Included among them are:

- carmustine
- lomustine
- semustine

The alkylating agents can cause leukemia, and one of them, cyclophosphamide, may cause bladder cancer.

That alkylating agents drugs may cause some other cancer is easy to understand. All of them fight cancer because they are toxic, or poisonous, to cells—and sometimes to healthy cells.

IMMUNOSUPPRESSIVE DRUGS

Immunosuppressive drugs are those used to fight an inflammatory process associated with some diseases. An inflammatory response occurs when, often for unknown reasons, the body's immune system becomes powerfully overactive, basically fighting its own cells. Some examples of diseases characterized by an inflammatory response are rheumatoid arthritis, systemic lupus erythematosus, and inflammatory bowel disease. They can cause devastating and debilitating symptoms when left untreated.

Some of the immunosuppressive drugs used to treat the symptoms of these diseases include imuran and cyclosporin. These medications can not only significantly improve quality of life, allowing people to live their life with less pain and handicapping symptoms, but may even save lives. They work by suppressing the body's immune system (hence their name). And that's exactly why they may cause cancer. Because they suppress the immune system, which is basically the body's surveillance system, the "cancer-patrolling" apparatus may also be suppressed. The most common associated cancer is lymphoma.

But it is crucial to keep perspective. Would someone with multiple myeloma, potentially a very lethal cancer, refuse treatment because of a small risk of developing leukemia some day? Would someone with rheumatoid arthritis let their disease progress to a stage requiring them to be wheelchair-bound because of a slight risk of developing lymphoma?

People must thoughtfully consider the risks, and realize they are overwhelmingly outweighed by the benefits of these drugs. An analogy is deciding whether to take a slow boat to China or fly—saving literally weeks of time. The risk of an airplane crash is definitely worth the benefit of the time saved. Overall, the gains in survival from cancer drugs far outweigh the associated risk of leukemia.

Doctors and researchers are continually looking to find the most therapeutic regimen for cancers and other diseases —one that also carries the lowest risk of side-effects, such as cancer. This reminds us of the importance of continually studying the effectiveness of drug therapy.

Predicting the Carcinogenicity of a Drug

Why don't we use animal studies to predict whether or not drugs, such as DES, will cause cancer in humans?

Some drugs cause cancer in animals, but not in man. An example is isoniazid, used to treat tuberculosis, which causes lung tumors in mice but not in rats or hamsters. When injected into rats, sodium penicillin causes sarcomas, but does not seem to be a cancer risk to humans. Hormones found in oral contraceptive pills have been known for years to cause liver cancer in laboratory animals. If we were to make judgments about the risk of a drug merely on the basis of the rat alone, the pill would never have been introduced. In many cases, the deaths caused by cancer-causing drugs could not have been predicted, and in that sense were unpreventable.

In the case of DES, there was obviously negligence on the part of some physicians who prescribed the drug during the 1960s—when it was clear that the drug did not decrease the risk of miscarriage. During this time, evidence was also mounting that hormones of any kind, taken in large doses, increased the risk of developing cancer. All that can be said is that some physicians, who for one reason or another did not keep up with the literature, were simply not well-enough informed.

In evaluating drugs, it seems that animal testing can only provide us with warnings. They cannot predict human carcinogenicity with any certainty. Decisions on the use of certain drugs have to depend on certain results of animal experiments—does the drug cause cancer in one species or several, and at one site or many? Decisions should also depend on analyses of the drug's chemical structure (does it resemble known carcinogens?), its purpose, and target population. Ultimately a drug's risks and benefits are ascertained by doing clinical trials in human beings.

How to Reduce Your Risk of Cancer

1. Never take any drug, whether prescription or over-the-counter, while pregnant without asking your doctor first.

2. Don't take any drug unnecessarily unless you're absolutely convinced you need it.

3. Choose your doctor carefully. If possible, choose one affiliated with a university or medical school—he or she will be more likely to keep up to date on the medical literature. Ultimately, you have to decide on drug usage based on the doctor's opinion, so you have to have confidence in his/her competence.

4. If you are not sure about the medication recommendations given you by one doctor, get an opinion from another doctor.

9

Occupation

In 1921, Phillip Hill, age twenty-three, began working at a dye manufacturing plant in New Jersey. In the course of his many tasks, he loaded vats with raw chemicals, operated machines and cleaned out the tanks once the processing was done. As a result he came in contact with a multitude of industrial chemicals.

Sometimes the fumes from the vats overwhelmed him. It was not unusual for his skin to come in contact with the various fluids he was mixing, as solutions seeped through his shirt and pants. During his twelve years at the plant, Phillip did not use any special type of protective clothing or equipment.

In 1933, he began to notice traces of blood in his urine. The blood appeared irregularly, present one day, and gone the next. Soon thereafter, he suffered noticeable weight loss, medium-grade fever, and tenderness in the area of his bladder. Urination became frequent and it was increasingly accompanied by a painful burning sensation. A cystoscopic examination, where a small tube was inserted into his urethra, revealed the presence of a large malignant tumor. Surgery was impractical. He died of industrially induced bladder cancer at the age of thirty-six.

*   *   *

Stuart Murphy was one of a few hundred men and women who joined in the shipbuilding effort at the Long Beach Naval Shipyard in 1942.

He helped install asbestos insulation in the steam power plants. As he described it, "You would take the white stuff, and make mud out of it, and throw it on the pipes."

Asbestos is an exceedingly dry mineral fiber, and working with it was often like being in the middle of a snowstorm. When conditions became particularly bad, Stuart would hold his breath as long as he could, but inevitably the asbestos cloud would outlast him, forcing him to breath deeply.

After working there for six months, Stuart quit, spent the next four years in the navy, returned to college and by 1950 was teaching high school physics in Chicago.

In 1966, twenty-four years after he spent six months at the shipyard, he experienced a persistent cough. He became breathless after walking up even one flight of stairs at school. Eventually, his breathing became so strained that he could be heard on the other side of the room.

An x-ray showed heavy shadows in the lower two-thirds of his lung field. Stuart's condition was diagnosed as diffuse pleural mesothelioma, a cancer usually caused by exposure to asbestos. His physician informed him that because the condition eventually covers the whole lung area, often spreading to the entire abdomen, surgery was impossible.

He could not remove all the damaged organs and still have a surviving patient. Stuart was dead within a year.

* * *

Marty Anderson joined the staff of a plastics manufacturing group in the midwestern United States in 1959, when he was twenty-two years old. He did not have any particular education or training, so he started at the bottom of the ladder, accepting an assignment as a "pot cleaner."

The plastic materials were made from a colorless gas called "vinyl chloride monomer" or VCM, a substance derived from chlorine and petroleum or natural gases. VCM is the raw material from which polyvinylchloride (PVC) resin is made during a process called polymerization. The resin is used to make plastic products. Once the vinyl chloride monomer was brought to the plant, it was unloaded, and piped in measured amounts into polymerization reactor vats. This was accomplished through an essentially closed system. Marty and his associates did not have to worry about coming into contact with VCM at that point. Then, catalysts, emulsifiers, and other chemicals were added to the VCM gas in the vat, heat and pressure applied, and the reaction carried out to its desired point.

After that, the polymerized material was dropped into a secondary vat and the VCM gas which had not reacted was recovered and recycled back through a closed system. The polymerized material then entered a third set of tanks from which it was dried and packaged. The end products in this third tank were three different materials: first the PVC resin, a powder of the texture of refined sugar; second, a PVC paste, a very fine powder with the texture of processed flour; and third, a PVC latex, a stable suspension of PVC in liquid.

Up until this point in the polymerization process, no one, including Marty, came in contact with large amounts of vinyl chloride monomer or any other chemical.

However, after the processing was complete, it was Marty's job, and that of the other pot cleaners, to open the reactor, climb into the six by ten foot tank, and with a hammer and chisel, chip the powder off the inside surface. Before he entered the tank, the air had been replaced a number of times, but nevertheless, when he opened the reactor it was not unusual for a burst of air, complete with particles of powder, to come in contact with his face momentarily. When he was in the tank doing his work, the only source of fresh air was a two-foot opening at the top. Sometimes as he chipped away at the powder, VCM gas trapped within the powder during polymerization was released.

The job was dull, always messy, and sometimes it became very hot in the plant. Frequently, Marty and his co-workers would take a break and cool off by throwing a cup or two of the vinyl chloride liquid on each others' backs. It evaporates quickly—it was like pouring ether on your skin, and the effect was refreshing.

Vinyl chloride is a colorless, faintly sweet-smelling gas at room temperature. Some of Marty's friends liked the sweet smell and the anaesthetic effect it had on them. They literally became hooked on the stuff and would sneak sniffs whenever they could.

Marty Anderson continued to work at the plant and in the mid-1960s was promoted to a more pleasant task.

He was in excellent health until 1973. Around that time, he noticed that his stools took on a tarlike shade of black.

He consulted a physician who made tentative diagnosis of "bleeding ulcer" and put him on a special diet.

But a few months later he returned, this time complaining of vague pain in the upper right quadrant of his body. A physical exam showed that his liver was markedly enlarged, and a subsequent liver scan found a large lesion on the left lobe. Exploratory surgery confirmed that Marty had angiosarcoma, an extremely rare liver cancer. He underwent cobalt treatment and after a stormy course recovered enough to return to work for a while. But in September of 1974, he succumbed to angiosarcoma, later to be linked to his PVC exposure. He was thirty-seven years old.

Occupational Illnesses

For centuries it has been known that certain occupations increase workers' risks of developing various diseases. Tragically, the association between the exposure and the risk was made after the fact, and human lives were lost.

The classic example of occupationally induced cancer was that reported by Percivall Pott in his book, *Chirurgical Observations,* which included a chapter entitled, "A Short Treatise of the Chimney Sweeper's Cancer." The chapter only contained 725 words, but the observations recorded in it provided the first clear description of an environmental cause of cancer, implied a way to prevent the disease and led indirectly to the synthesis of the first known pure carcinogen. He described the plight of the chimney sweeps as follows:

> The fate of these people seems singularly hard; in their infancy, they are most frequently treated with great

brutality, and almost starved with cold and hunger; they are thrust up narrow, and sometimes hot chimneys, where they are bruised, burned, and almost suffocated; and when they get to puberty, become liable to a noisome, painful, and fatal disease.

As Pott alluded, the sweeps were young boys who were kept on a minimal diet in an effort to keep them small, so they could physically enter the chimneys and do their most unpleasant task. Hygiene was very poor and in the course of their sweeping, soot accumulated on their scrotums. Pott had identified an environmental cause of scrotal cancer. In 1915, Japanese workers, Yamagiwa and Ichikawa, supplied another part of the answer: they painted coal tar on a rabbit's ear and produced cancer. And in 1933, Cook and his associates put together the last piece of the puzzle: they identified the powerful carcinogen benzo(a)pyrene from coal tar.

The list of occupational cancer hazards is long and depressing, as is the list of occupations known or suspected to increase the risk of contracting cancer (see Tables 1-3). The cases of the dial workers and early radiologists who succumbed to the hazards of their trade, for example, have already been mentioned.

But there are many more examples: vineyard workers using arsenic sprays; smelters and others who came in frequent contact with high levels of inorganic arsenic, manifest high rates of skin, lung, and liver cancers; shoemakers, who worked with a solvent containing a high percentage of benzene, had a very high rate of leukemia. Members of the chromate industry had unusually high rates for cancers of the lung, nasal cavity, sinuses, and larynx. Workers coming in frequent contact with mustard gas had significantly higher mortality from cancers of the larynx, lung, trachea, and bronchi than most men. And the list goes on.

Occupationally induced diseases are sometimes rather difficult to identify. With ten or more years elapsing between exposure and the onset of symptoms of disease, the victim may be in a job different from the one that originally exposed him/her to the diseases.

Asbestos—"The Magic Mineral"

Because it has so many useful chemical and physical properties, asbestos was at one time called the "magic mineral." Besides being able to withstand temperatures of over 500°C (932°F), asbestos does not react to many acids and other chemicals and is a good heat and sound insulator. This combination of characteristics makes it extremely versatile, and it has been used in various products for over 4,500 years.

Asbestos is actually the name of a collection of minerals that share the same properties. The most commonly encountered forms are chrysotile ("white asbestos") and amosite ("blue asbestos"). Each type has its own characteristics that make it more or less suitable for a given use, and each may have a different degree of health risk. More than 90 percent of all asbestos used is chrysotile.

One of the early uses of asbestos was to make fireproof curtains in theaters, after a series of fires in the gas-lit theaters of the 1800s killed hundreds of people. Its use in the ships built during World War II was a critical and useful part of the war effort. Applied to structural steelwork of large building, asbestos prevents the heat of a fire from weakening the girders, which would otherwise result in the collapse of the building.

Even today, despite the concern over its potential to cause disease, asbestos is contained in many products. Textiles, paper, ropes, wicks, stoves, filters, floor tiles, roofing shingles, clutch facings, waterpipe, cements, fillers, felt, fireproof clothing, gaskets, battery boxes, clapboard, wallboard, firedoors, fire curtains, and brake linings may contain asbestos in varying amounts.

The Flawed Miracle

One of the earliest studies documenting a hazard to humans from asbestos was published in 1900, when Dr. H. Montague Murray described pulmonary fibrosis at autopsy in a worker employed fourteen years previously in an asbestos textile factory. W. E. Cooke, writing in a British medical journal in 1927, gave the name "asbestosis" to Dr. Murray's pulmonary fibrosis. British experts surveyed mill employees in an asbestos textile operation in 1929 and recommended methods to reduce employee exposure to the dust. Optimistically, they predicted that "the outlook . . . is good. In the space of a decade or thereabouts, the effect of energetic application of preventive measures should be apparent in a great reduction in the incidence of fibrosis."

While the incidence of fibrosis did go down, the first report of lung cancer in an asbestos worker was published in 1935. However, it was not until a large-scale study of insulation workers was published in 1964 that the association between asbestosis and bronchogenic carcinoma (a type of lung cancer) was suggested in workers using products containing asbestos. Mesothelioma, a rare tumor of the lining of the abdomen or chest, was reported in South Africa in 1960 among people exposed to certain types of asbestos. Whether asbestos is the sole cause of mesothelioma is unclear, because prior exposure cannot be confirmed in all cases of mesothelioma, and other substances have had similar effects in laboratory studies.

It was not until the late 1960s that it was realized that indirect exposure to asbestos may also cause disease. Employees of the Devonport Dockyard in England were surveyed, and asbestos-related diseases were documented in workers other than the insulators who had worked directly with asbestos. Some English shipyard workers became ill with increasing frequency in the 1960s, after a twenty-five- to thirty-year latency period between first exposure to asbestos and clinical symptoms. In 1965 it became apparent that living near an asbestos factory or sharing a home with an asbestos worker might cause asbestos-related disease. This was confirmed by another study in 1975.

There is, however, very little—if any—risk to occupants of buildings in which there are traces of asbestos. In 1991, The American Medical Association's Council on Scientific Affairs said in their position paper on the topic that asbestos risk has been greatly inflated: "Contrary to what was described as public misconception: asbestos posed far less risk to the health of the everyday occupants of buildings than that posed by smoking, drug and alcohol abuse, improper diet and lack of exercise."

How Does Asbestos Cause Disease?

The overwhelming majority of asbestos-caused disease occurs from occupational exposure—prolonged exposure at relatively high levels—to amphibole-type asbestos. Such asbestos exposure can cause four diseases: asbestosis, lung cancer, mesothelioma, and pleural disease.

Asbestos-related diseases occur after a relatively long latent period, or a lag from time of exposure to onset of symptoms (four to seven years for fibrosis; twenty to forty for cancers). It is also crucial to remember that critical concentration: nearly all asbestos-related disease occurs in workers who are exposed to asbestos levels several thousand times higher than those found inside commercial, residential and school buildings. Linda Fisher of the EPA's Office of Pesticides and Toxic Substances explains:

> The mere presence of a hazardous substance, such as asbestos on an auditorium ceiling, no more implies disease than a potential poison in a medicine cabinet or under a kitchen sink implies poisoning. Asbestos fibers must be released from the material in which they are contained, and an individual must breathe those fibers in order to incur any chance of disease.

Asbestos and Lung Cancer

Asbestos generally does not cause cancer by itself, but acts to help, or promote, other substances in causing cancer. The primary carcinogenic agent in most asbestos-related lung cancers is cigarette smoke. In fact, asbestos workers who smoke are over fifty times more likely to get lung cancer than asbestos workers who do not smoke, according to a major investigation involving over 17,000 asbestos insulation workers. Smoking asbestos workers are ninety times more likely to get lung cancer than nonexposed nonsmokers. In stark contrast, asbestos workers who do not smoke are only 5 times more likely to die from lung cancer than are nonexposed nonsmokers. Past occupational exposure to asbestos accounts for about four thousand to six thousand cases of lung cancer per year.

A synergistic effect of cigarette smoking has also been demonstrated for deaths due to asbestosis, or fibrotic lung disease. Both obstructive lung disease caused by smoking and restrictive lung disease caused by asbestos exposure can coexist within the same lung, leading to a greater degree of disability than would occur in the presence of only one of the factors. Thus, a cigarette smoker may die as a result of a degree of fibrosis that would not be fatal in a nonsmoker.

How much asbestos is necessary to cause lung cancer? While some scientists insist that even a single fiber can cause cancer, a look at the levels of asbestos in the air we breathe and the water we drink suggests otherwise. At the same time, though, there is no information on exactly what level of asbestos causes health problems. But occupational health experts, in the 1990s, do believe that present levels of asbestos allowed in workplaces are safe and not expected to produce any measurable impairment.

Were Asbestos-related Deaths Preventable?

The evidence that asbestos inhalation posed a serious hazard to human health accumulated very slowly during the first half of this century. It is easy to see how a nation at war, in desperate need of well-equipped ships, would put worker protection devices on a low priority, especially since they had no real reason to believe that working with asbestos posed a problem.

But with the accumulation of evidence throughout the 1950s and 1960s, it is more difficult to understand why the problem was not taken more seriously later. Many of the larger asbestos plants instituted protective measures in the 1950s. But some of the smaller ones were evidently very careless about human exposure to this known cancer-causing agent. A particularly infamous example was a plant in Tyler, Texas, which as late as 1970 was exposing its workers to asbestos levels sixty times, or more, higher than the currently accepted level.

It seems that many of the earlier deaths were not preventable, in the sense that knowledge was so incomplete that a health risk was not recognized. But many asbestos plants were negligently slow in correcting matters—at the cost of the lives of many of their workers. The workers themselves, in some instances, often did not act to protect their own health, refusing to use the protective masks that were supplied.

Today, industrial levels of asbestos are under strict government regulations, the limit in the plants being two fibers per cubic centimeter of air, where in early decades it often got as high as two hundred, three hundred, or more per cubic centimeter of air. We can pinpoint some populations with a high risk of cancer from past asbestos exposure—asbestos products workers and insulators who were exposed before adequate controls were in effect are still clearly high-risk populations. Others who might still be working under high-risk conditions are those employed at smaller plants, where controls are often less rigorous. Efforts to prevent disease in these populations would be an important public service to them.

Asbestos and the General Public

One of the most frightening aspects of the asbestos story is the fact that the deaths recorded were not limited to one job category in one type of workplace. There were many women who became victims of mesothelioma apparently simply because they regularly washed their asbestos-worker-husband's clothes; men and women who became victims because, as children, they played in a field contaminated with asbestos dust.

There is no doubt that asbestos is a frightening substance. Workers must be protected from its effects, and we have to do all we can to reduce its presence in ambient air. For instance, building demolition—which frees asbestos fibers in their dry form, one in which they are easily inhaled—should be strictly controlled.

Asbestos in the Schools

Schools built or renovated from 1940 to 1973 were required to have asbestos insulation as a fire safety measure. Besides this sprayed insulation, asbestos has been used in such materials as acoustical insulation, cement products, plaster, fireproof textiles, vinyl floor tiles and thermal insulation. As long as the material is intact, there appears to be no need for concern.

The asbestos danger arises when damage from ordinary wear-and-tear, vandalism, or water makes the material *friable*. This means that it can be easily crumbled, pulverized or reduced to powder in the hand, and hence it may be capable of releasing fibers. It is important to note that not all friable materials contain asbestos. Microscopic or chemical testing and studies on crystalline structure are necessary to confirm that the friable material is indeed asbestos.

Unfortunately, the EPA does not suggest any concrete guidelines. Schools have been the central focus of the asbestos panic.

The EPA first required that all schools inspect for friable (easily crumbled) asbestos in May 1982, with the passage of the Asbestos-In-Schools Identification and Notification Rule. This rule also called for parent, teacher, and school worker notification.

In 1984, Congress passed the Asbestos School Hazard Abatement Act (ASHAA) to provide financial assistance to those schools with serious asbestos hazards and concurrent financial need. From 1985 to late 1991, the ASHAA program provided approximately $291 million to more than 1,100 needy school districts and private schools. ASHAA was reauthorized in 1990, calling for revisions to its accreditation plan, which, among other things, would increase training requirements for abatement workers.

On October 22, 1986, President Reagan authorized the Asbestos Hazard Emergency Response Act (AHERA), taking the asbestos issue in schools two steps further. All public and private schools were thus required to inspect for asbestos, develop asbestos management plans and submit them to the state, and then implement appropriate response actions called abatement. Abatement could be in-place management, repair, encapsulation, or removal. AHERA required that all inspection and abatement, mandated to begin by July 1988 in every school judged to be unsafe, be carried out by accredited personnel.

In 1990, the National School Boards Association estimated the cost of abatement work in public schools alone at more than $6 billion, only a portion of which has been or will be paid for by the federal government. The EPA itself estimated the cost of removing asbestos from all public and commercial buildings at $51 billion.

It is critical to keep a perspective on the amount of asbestos in schools. At no time were children thought to be exposed to health-threatening amounts of asbestos. The average level of asbestos in schools was just 0.0007 fibers per ml, which is nearly three thousand times less than the legal amount allowed by OSHA in workplaces using asbestos (where workers are exposed for eight hours each day, five days per week).

It is also crucial to remember that abatement doesn't always mean removal; it is just one option. EPA's Linda Fisher, in fact, told the U.S. House of Representatives:

> It bears repeating that, for most situations, EPA under the AHERA program does not mandate removal of asbestos. . . . In addition, removal is often not a school district's or other building owner's best course of action to reduce asbestos exposure. In fact, an improper removal can create

a dangerous situation where none previously existed. Instead of removal, a conscientious in-place management program will usually control fiber releases, particularly when the materials are not significantly damaged or are not likely to be disturbed. *EPA does recommend in-place management whenever asbestos is discovered.*

The American Medical Association agreed with this line of thinking, recommending removal only when damage to the asbestos-containing material is severe and cannot be repaired, or when there might be a significant release of fibers during building renovation or demolition.

Maintaining friable asbestos in place is not only the wisest choice from a health standpoint, but it is also the easiest and most inexpensive way to manage asbestos. *Money* magazine estimated in 1987 that the cost of maintaining asbestos in place in the average home is approximately $10 to $50, whereas removal can cost up to $5,000.

It bears repeating again that just because asbestos is present, there isn't necessarily a health hazard. Concern about the presence of asbestos arises only when the asbestos fibers are released into the air (such as when asbestos-containing materials become damaged) in sufficiently dangerous quantities and are subsequently inhaled.

Vinyl Chloride

Polymerization of the vinyl chloride monomer began in Germany in 1939. The United States became involved in its production some five years later. Polyvinyl chloride, much like asbestos, was hailed as a miracle substance: cheap, stable, fire resistant, and able to assume an extraordinary range of soft and hard forms. Immediately, it was designated for possible use in floor tiles, medical supplies, phonograph records, auto seat covers, wire insulation, and for many other purposes.

Was it safe? During the 1940s, everyone seemed to think so. The primary worry then was the fire explosion potential of the gas. Once that was under control, the concerns were minimal.

In 1949, ten years after it was discovered, a Russian report indicated that a hepatitis-like condition occurred in more than 25 percent of seventy-three polyvinyl chloride workers examined. The results of the report were circulated, but no one was terribly alarmed. During the 1950s, there were reports in many countries of a vaguely defined "vinyl chloride disease," the characteristics of which were nausea, dizziness, and sometimes temporary loss of consciousness. Somewhat later came reports of a thickening of the skin at the fingertips, gradual dissolution of bone calcium at the fingertips, and heightened sensitivity to cold (collectively known as acro-osteolysis), in a small proportion of the workers involved in the manual cleaning of PVC reactors.

Also during the 1950s, there were scattered industry-sponsored animal experiments suggesting that the vinyl chloride monomer, in high doses, might have some toxic effects—possibly affecting the liver. As a result, in the early 1960s, the American Conference of Governmental Industrial Hygienists, a voluntary standard-setting organization, put the maximum safe exposure level for workers at 500 parts per million (ppm). Dow Chemical thought even that figure was too high. When a 1961 animal experiment showed adverse liver effects (but no cancer) in animals at doses as low as 100 ppm, they put an upper exposure limit at their plant at 50 ppm.

The reports of the local bone and skin reactions (acro-osteolysis) among a small number of pot cleaners led industry to do away with the manual mechanism of pot cleaning. In the late 1960s, high-pressure water hoses for cleaning were introduced, and only in rare cases did men ever climb into the tanks again.

There was some concern about potential ill effects of some aspects of the plastics production mechanism, so industry scientists made a voluntary commitment to keep testing vinyl chloride.

In May of 1970, at the 10th International Cancer Congress in Houston, Texas, Dr. P.L. Viola of the Regina Elena Institute for Cancer Research in Rome, and a medical director of Solvay and Cie, a leading European PVC producer, reported that cancers (but not angiosarcoma) in test animals could be produced at extremely high levels of exposure to vinyl chloride (10,000 to 30,000 ppm). Dr. Viola concluded that there was "no implication to human pathology" from this experiment, and no need to be concerned about workers exposed to less than 500 ppm of the vinyl chloride monomer. At that point, most PVC plants in the United States were well below that level anyway.

In March of 1972, still eager to collect more data, seventeen U.S. manufacturers of PVC and the VCM agreed to sponsor both animal experiments and health studies on vinyl chloride monomer workers in this country, the studies to be administered by the Manufacturing Chemists Association (now the Chemical Manufacturer's Association). At the same time, the European industries were sponsoring similar animal tests, under the direction of Dr. Cesare Maltoni of the Institute di Oncologia and Certro Tumor in Bologna, Italy.

In January 1973, Dr. Maltoni came up with some disturbing results. He detected a variety of tumors (including liver tumors) in test animals subjected to concentrations of VCM as low as 250 ppm. In November 1973, Dr. Viola, who had previously been able to show malignant tumors at very high levels, confirmed that they could be induced at 250 ppm. The interest in the possible ill effects of vinyl chloride became more intense. But there was still no reason to believe that human health was threatened, even at high levels of exposure to the monomer.

Then, in late 1973, Dr. John L. Creech, a local Louisville surgeon who helped oversee the health of B.F. Goodrich workers, casually mentioned to the Goodrich plant physician, Dr. Maurice N. Johnson, that he had recently seen two cases of a rare disease—angiosarcoma of the liver—one earlier that year and one about two years before. Dr. Johnson was startled, for he recognized this to be the same type of tumor that had been reported to occur in the Maltoni rat study. Angiosarcoma of the liver is very rare, only some twenty-five to thirty cases being diagnosed each year in the U.S. When a third Louisville case of angiosarcoma came to their attention a few weeks later, they realized it was no coincidence.

On January 22, 1974, the B.F. Goodrich Company notified employees, the National Institute of Occupational Safety and Health, and the Kentucky State Department of Labor that three of its workers had died from angiosarcoma of the liver.

This link was made by two astute physicians, who, knowing that angiosarcoma was an extremely rare disease, concluded that there was some causal significance. Needless to say, if vinyl chloride caused a common tumor such as lung cancer, the picture would have been much less clear-cut and would have required many more cases and much more elaborate epidemiological manipulation to associate the tumor with the industrial exposure.

After the initial announcement, vinyl chloride plants outside Louisville began to examine their death record over the past ten years. Sometimes the cause of death was listed "primarily liver cancer" or "liver cirrhosis" but eventually it was established that the more likely cause was a liver angiosarcoma.

Within weeks of the discovery of the human cancer, Professor Maltoni of Rome found that tumors could be induced in animals at 50 ppm. But people hardly needed any more convincing then.

Even prior to the findings that the vinyl chloride monomer could cause cancer in workers exposed to high levels of it (note here that it is the monomer, or VCM, not the plastic resin, or PVC, that was linked to both human and animal tumors) federal regulatory agencies took action against the chemical. In 1973 and 1974 they banned various aerosol sprays containing the monomer as a propellant. Similarly, when it was found that traces of the VCM could migrate from plastic liquor bottles to the alcohol, the government banned PVC plastic bottles for this use (the primary concern was that the taste of the liquor would be affected). Ironically, not only were the VCM levels migrating to alcohol very small, but they would most likely have completely evaporated before the consumer had completed mixing his or her drink.

There was no reason to believe that either the aerosols or the use of VCM in the manufacture of liquor bottles ever posed any hazard whatsoever to human health, but in the interest of complete safety, the withdrawals were made. The industry did not oppose either move.

There has been no further concern shown by either the EPA or OSHA since 1974 about the adequacy of the existing regulations to protect both workers and the general public.

Could It Have Been Prevented?

With the state of technology available throughout the 1940s and 1950s, there was no way that scientists could have known that intense exposure to vinyl chloride monomer would cause human cancer. The moment that industry scientists became even slightly suspicious, protective measures were instituted and worker exposure levels drastically lowered.

Although the animal experiments of the 1940s and 1950s were interesting, they were not alarming, by any means. Many different chemicals, industrial or natural will increase the chance of tumors forming in test animals. When early animal tests suggested that VCM in high doses might be harmful, the manufacturers did the only thing they could do—reduce worker exposure levels and keep testing.

Indeed, if you compare the vinyl chloride story to that of asbestos, you have a case of excellent industrial surveillance. Mount Sinai's Dr. Irving Selikoff calls the vinyl chloride incident a "success story": "a success for science having defined the problem; a success for labor in the rapid mobilization of concern; success for government in urgently collecting data, evaluating and translating it into necessary regulations; and success for industry in preparing the necessary engineering controls to minimize or eliminate the hazard."

Indeed, it was industry that supported all the studies. Ralph L. Harding, Jr., President of the Society of the Plastics Industry, Inc., summarized it: "This is a unique situation. Industry financed the studies and industry blew the whistle on itself." But this fact is often quickly forgotten by those who want to pin what was in most respects an unavoidable tragedy on "evil industry."

PVC and VCM and the Public

The vinyl chloride episode was another frightening case of occupational disease, but again, it is easy to panic and lose perspective.

All authenticated cases of angiosarcoma occurred among workers engaged in closed environments during the conversion process (Polymerization) of the *vinyl chloride monomer* to polyvinyl chloride resin or in workers directly handling the monomer. A variety of estimates put the minimal amount of exposure leading to disease at between 200 and 500 ppm—probably more. The average length of worker exposure was seventeen years: the shortest four years. This was an exposure of eight hours a day, five days a week, for 50 weeks a year to significantly higher levels than are currently allowed. The chances of a member of the general public being exposed to significant amounts of vinyl chloride monomer with the new, very low standards, are almost nil.

Although press reports indicate otherwise, a government survey of angiosarcoma deaths in the U.S. between 1964 and 1974 concluded that there was "no evidence that living around a vinyl chloride plant is a risk factor in the occurrence of liver angiosarcoma." This conclusion has been confirmed in more recent studies.

Prior to the disclosure that a small number of workers exposed to VCM had developed a rare form of liver cancer, the plastic industry did a significant amount of research to ensure that even small amounts of the vinyl chloride monomer were not present in wraps that contact food. During the 1960s, and for the first couple of years in the 1970s, trace amounts of the monomer were detected in some food wraps. Although the quantity was most certainly not enough to cause any harm, their mere presence raised eyebrows at the Food and Drug Administration. Our current laws state that substances that may migrate to foods from wrapping (thus termed intentionally added food additives) are illegal if shown to cause cancer (in any amount under any circumstances) in animals.

As of now, there is no significant risk posed to the individual who uses plastic wrap or plastic containers.

Simply because intense levels of exposure to the vinyl chloride *monomer* increased risks of this rare form of liver cancer among plant workers does not mean that the PVC resin is cancer-causing. Even more important, the plastic products themselves that are many stages removed from the monomer and PVC resin—for instance, automobile seats and phonograph records—pose no health threat. The "new car smell," for instance, has nothing to do with VCM or PVC.

Application of heat to plastic products does not lead to the depolymerization of the PVC back to the chloride gas. When PVC is burned, some toxic gases are given off, most notably phosgene and hydrochloric acid. Recently, certain consumer groups have raised questions about the safety of PVC tubing to hold electrical wires in the New York City subway system. Despite unanswered questions about whether burning PVC is any more dangerous than burning wood and other ordinary combustibles, the authorities decided to remove the PVC tubing and replace it with steel conduit. A great deal more research on fire deaths needs to be done to determine if the use of PVC is an increased fire hazard or not. Currently, only carbon monoxide is routinely assayed in autopsies of fire victims; more sophisticated studies are necessary to settle this issue.

Other Occupational Cancers

In addition to asbestos and polyvinyl chloride, there are around 30 substances identified that have caused cancer at higher, occupational exposures. For example, benzene at industrial levels of exposure causes leukemia. Dimethyl formamide, a chemical used in several industries, including leather tanning and fighter jet maintenance, has been implicated as a cause of testicular cancer. Refer to tables 1–5 for a summary of this information.

How Frequently Do Occupational Cancers Occur?

Most epidemiologists agree that it is very difficult to estimate the percentage of future cancers that might be accounted for by occupational exposure. During the late 1970s a number of distinguished researchers, including Dr. John Higginson, came up with a ball-park estimate in the range of 3 to 5 percent. Another epidemiologist went so far as to set 10 percent as a possible upper limit.

But commencing in 1978, following the release of a draft

of a controversial paper on the subject (see below), there has been a heated debate among public health professionals about the exact extent of occupational cancers. In 1993, the 3 to 5 percent estimate seems to be in favor, with the larger percentages seriously in doubt. The so-called "Estimates" paper described below is an example of what happens when science and politics mix, and only serve to blur what is already a difficult issue.

The OSHA Paper—
Califano's Curious Cancer Estimates

In September 1978, Joseph A. Califano, Jr., then Secretary of Health, Education and Welfare, told an AFL-CIO conference on occupational safety and health, "At least 20 percent of all cancer in the United States—and perhaps more—may be work-related. . . . It is estimated that 10 to 15 percent of all cancer deaths in the United States each year will be associated with previous exposure to asbestos."

Mr. Califano's numbers came from a draft report, "Estimates of the Fraction of Cancer in the United States Related to Occupational Factors," dated September 15, 1978. According to its title page, the report was "prepared by the National Cancer Institute (NCI), the National Institute of Environmental Health Science (NIEHS), the National Institute of Occupational Safety and Health (NIOSH)." Ten "contributors" were listed in alphabetical order with their institutional affiliation: Dr. Kenneth Bridbord, NIOSH; Dr. Pierre Decoufle, NCI; Dr. Joseph F. Fraumeni, Jr., NCI; Dr. David G. Hoel, NIESH; Dr. Robert N. Hoover, NCI; Dr. David P. Rall, director NIESH; Dr. Umberto Saffioti, NCI; Dr. Marvin A. Schneiderman, NCI;

and Dr. Arthur C. Upton, director, NCI. Dr. Nicholas Day, NCI, is listed as a contributor to the appendix. All were prominent, highly respected scientists.

Although this paper is over fifteen years old, we are still seeing its repercussions. Its unrealistically high cancer figures were quoted with disturbing regularity in federal policy documents for many years. For example, a Toxic Substances Strategy Committee report to the president of May 1980 based its cancer prevention policy on these estimates.

Mr. Califano's estimates were alarming, especially when one considers that the accepted estimate for industrially induced cancers is 3 to 7 percent. Although the paper was widely publicized, it was harshly criticized in the scientific community. Sir Richard Doll, perhaps the world's foremost epidemiologist, said of the Estimates papers: "I regard it as scientific nonsense." Most telling was the fact that the paper was never published in a scientific journal.

From where did this paper originate? In 1977, these men had formed a group to look at occupational factors related to cancer. They felt that previous estimates to look at these relationships were inadequate. (Previous attempts had tried to assign a single cause to each cancer.) The group wanted to emphasize the importance of another approach to cancer causality: that cancer is a disease with multiple stages and multiple causes. A cancer might start with a single cell that becomes cancerous from some cause, genetic or environmental (and environmental means all aspects of life, including diet, smoking, alcohol, the surrounding air, sunlight, and background radiation, as well as occupation). The cancer may then be stimulated, or inhibited, by factors other than the original one at any stage until a tumor actually appears.

Lung cancer in asbestos workers is an example of the

way one cause may stimulate or enhance another; asbestos workers who smoke have a far greater risk of developing lung cancer than asbestos workers who don't smoke.

The National Institute of Health group had focused on occupationally related cancers for a second reason: the Occupational Safety and Health Administration (OSHA) was planning a hearing on the topic. In the summer of 1978, after the group had been meeting irregularly for the most of one year, NCI was asked to prepare testimony for the OSHA hearing to rebut American industry's estimate that only one percent of cancer is work-related. The group's pace suddenly quickened. The impression conveyed was one of frantic phone calls to consult vacationing group members, hasty editing, and the submission of the report to OSHA.

However, several contributors to the "Estimates" have said they thought the report was misused as a basis for policy planning. Clearly it didn't warrant the degree of confidence it received from federal regulatory agencies—"estimates" should not be used as a basis for regulation.

Perhaps the most insightful comment was made by then National Academy of Sciences president, Dr. Philip Handler at the dedication of the Northwestern University Cancer Center in May 1979: "What seems lost on some who would participate in the debate on the place of technology in our society, particularly those concerned with possible environmental carcinogenesis . . . is that the necessity for scientific rigor is even greater when scientific evidence is being offered as the basis for formulation of public policy than when it is simply expected to find its way into the marketplace of accepted scientific understanding. Science itself can benefit from early publication of properly documented preliminary findings. But surely public policy should not rest on observations so preliminary that they could not find acceptance for publication in an edited scientific journal."

Occupational Cancer: A Perspective

We have learned a great deal about occupational cancers in the past four decades. But the subject is still relatively new, and we are still groping with means to handle these types of cancers. On one hand some people maintain that human life is more important than any industry or product, and if a problem comes up, the item or items should be banned. On the other hand, other individuals, while agreeing that the protection of human life is the number one priority, point out there are safe ways of using unsafe materials and that we could institute effective protective measures for exposed workers, and base our actions and consider the issue in terms of six general guidelines. We must also remember that hastily chosen substitutes could be even more dangerous.

First, it is acknowledged that under some circumstances, high levels of occupational chemical exposure can cause cancer. Occupational studies have been very useful in identifying the potential carcinogenicity of chemicals because these groups of subjects are well defined and relatively easy to follow-up. However, the fact that a chemical causes cancer in an occupational setting at high doses does not automatically mean that traces or even low amounts of them also pose a risk. Certainly the fact that a human carcinogen shows up in some aspects of our environment should stimulate action. For instance, when asbestos traces were found in the water supply of Duluth, Minnesota, and New Orleans, that was a source of legitimate concern, even though we have no reason to believe that small amounts of ingested asbestos would have anything like the effects of high levels of inhaled asbestos. Nevertheless, it is something that should be investigated, and steps should be taken to reduce exposure as much as possible.

Second, it is critical in discussing occupational disease, that we not exaggerate the situation. In total, fewer than 100 workers have thus far been diagnosed as having VCM-induced angiosarcoma of the liver. But given the headline space the topic has been given, many people think the number is more like thirty thousand. This is not to minimize the tragedy of the men and women who were involved. It is to lend some perspective to the extent of the problem we are dealing with

Third, the chemicals we have discussed in this chapter pose, except in some very rare circumstances, a negligible risk to you unless you are working in an industrial situation that puts you in frequent contact with the chemicals. Worker populations may be small in comparison to the entire United States population, but they suffer much higher risks of cancer from exposure to some chemicals. However, these risks are small in comparison to the risk of lung cancer in a heavy smoker.

Fourth, most diseases identified with industrial causes are also caused by other factors. For instance, lung cancer risk is increased with exposure to asbestos. But many people associated with the asbestos business or living in an area near an asbestos plant die from lung cancer because they smoke cigarettes, not because of exposure to the fiber. Some workers in the chemical industry, and those living in the immediate vicinity, develop bladder tumors spontaneously, as a result of cigarette smoking, not because of occupational carcinogens. Angiosarcoma is such a rare disease that the analogy is not as appropriate here, but even in this case, rare liver disturbances do occur outside an occupational setting. In the months following the disclosure of the Goodrich VCM worker deaths, there were scattered reports of angiosarcoma of the liver in areas near the plant. Subsequent investigations indicated that these had nothing to do with polymerization of plastic materials, but were instead the results of better diagnosis; that is, with angiosarcoma in the newspapers constantly, physicians became more familiar with its symptoms and where, under other circumstances, they might have listed a cause of death as "liver cancer," they were then more specific.

Fifth, although tragedies have been associated with certain occupational chemicals, we can't forget that many of these very same chemicals have saved more lives than they have taken. For instance, in the furor over asbestos, many people forget that the "miracle fiber" was used to prevent fires and to make auto brakes safer. In discussing the much-maligned plastics, one cannot overlook its indispensable use in the medical field—blood bags and medical tubing that have saved thousands of lives. On another level, we have to remember that banning plastic bottles because of some hypothetical cancer risk will inevitably lead to more home accidents, some quite serious, maybe even fatal, from broken glass.

Sixth, we are not dealing with an "us versus them" situation. When it comes to industrial production in the United States, we are all in this together. We all benefit from the lifesaving and simply pleasurable aspects of modern living. While federal regulation and surveillance of employee working conditions in chemical plants—and in work environments that use chemicals—is obviously necessary, it is pointless to accuse an industry of deliberately using human life to their own advantage in making profits. That is an accusation more appropriate to the early part of this century, not the 1990s. On the other hand, it is clear that there is an ongoing need for monitoring the various chemical industries to ensure that established regulations are followed and that workers' health is not impaired by exposure to toxic or carcinogenic chemicals.

How to Reduce Your Risk of Cancer

1. If you work in a chemical plant, or in an environment in which you are exposed to industrial chemicals, always follow the safety instructions of your plant. At least some of the occupational tragedies of the past were due to workers being careless about their health.

2. Be extremely cautious when tearing down parts of a house or the structures that could be lined with asbestos. Be particularly careful when you encounter insulation material that may contain significant amounts of dry asbestos. Keep asbestos-containing materials wet, and wear a particle respirator when removing this material. Afterwards, place the mask and the waste in a plastic bag and throw it away. Or better yet, hire one of the many companies specializing in safe asbestos removal.

3. Stop smoking. Aside from the increased risk of cancer from the tobacco itself, there is synergism between the tobacco carcinogens and any other cancer-causing elements you may be exposed to. This means that the car-

cinogens from tobacco and any other source work together to significantly increase one's chance of developing cancer. This greatly increases your risk of contracting cancer far beyond what any one factor alone would.

Table 9.1
Occupational Exposures and
Their Associated Cancers

Wood dust	stomach, lung
Gasoline	stomach
Synthetic fibers	colorectum
Silica dust	lung (nonadenocarcinoma)
Mineral spirits	lung (squamous cell)
Gasoline exhaust & diesel exhaust	lung (squamous cell)
Cutting fluids	bladder
Aviation gasoline	kidney

Source: J. Siemiatycki, "Discovering Occupational Carcinogens in Population-based Case-Control Studies: Review of Findings from an Exposure-Based Approach and a Methodologic Comparison of Alternative Data Collection Strategies," *Recent Results in Cancer Research* 120 (1990): 25–38.

Table 9.2
Occupations at Risk for Bladder Cancer*

Petroleum workers
Machinists
Engineers
Truck drivers
Garage and gas station workers
Food counter workers
Cooks
Textile workers
Printers
Leather workers
Rubber workers
Dyestuff workers
Gas workers

Source: P. Vineis and L. Simonato. "Proportion of Lung and Bladder Cancers in Males Resulting from Occupation: A Systematic Approach," *Archives of Environmental Health* 46 (1991): 6.
*Review of 18 studies showed proportion of bladder cancers attributable to occupation to be from 0–2% to 24%.

Table 9.3
Occupations at Risk for Lung Cancer*

Arsenic producers
Vineyard workers
Roofers/asphalt workers
Coke plant workers
Gas workers
Producers of asbestos goods
Construction workers (insulation)
Shipyard and dockyard workers
Miners of arsenic, iron ore, asbestos, uranium/radon
Producers of bischloro-methylether, chloromethyl-methylether and chromate
    pigments
Producers of batteries
Cadmium and copper smelters
Chromium platers
Ferrochromium produers
Stell producers
Nickel refiners
Iron foundry workers
Producers of mustard gas
Asbestos exposure related-steamfitters, boilermakers, pipefitters, locomotive
    builders and repair workers, automobile brake workers

Source: P. Vineis and L. Simonato, "Proportion of Lung and Bladder Cancers in
    Males Resulting from Occupation: A Systematic Approach," *Archives of
    Environmental Health* 46: 6–15.
*Review of 16 papers (20 studies) showed proportion of lung cancers attributa-
    ble to occupation to be from 1% to 40%.

Table 9.4
Cancer Sites for Which Relationships with Occupational Exposures are Well-Established in Human Studies*

Site	Agent or Industrial Process	References
Bladder	Benzidine B-naphthylamine 4-Aminobiphenyl (xenyla-mine)	Rhen 1895; Ferguson et al., 1934; Case et al., 1954; Melick et al., 1955, Vigliani and Barsotti, 1961; Lieben, 1963; Goldwater et al., 1965; Mancuso and El-Attar, 1967; Melick et al., 1971; Zavon et al., 1973; Tsuchiya et al., 1975.
	Manufacture of certain dyes (e.g., auramine and magenta)	Case and Pearson, 1954.
	Gas retorts	Doll et al, 1965; Doll et al., 1972.
	Rubber and cable-making industries	Case and Hosker, 1954; Davies, 1965.
Blood (leukemia)	Benzene	Girard et al., 1971; Aksoy et al., 1974; Vigliani, 1976; Infante et al., 1977.
	X-radiation	Warren, 1956; Seltser and Sartwell, 1965; Warren and Lombard, 1966; Matanoski, et al., 1975.
Bone	Radium, Mesothorium	Martland, 1931; Polednak et al., 1978.
Larynx	Ethanol (ethyl alcohol) manufacture by strong acid (process diethyl sulfate)	Lynch et al., 1979.
	Isopropyl alcohol manufacture by strong acid process (diisopropyl sulfate)	Weil et al., 1952; Eckardt, 1974.
	Mustard gas	Wada et al., 1968.
Liver (Angiosarcoma)	Arsenic (inorganic compounds)	Roth, 1958.
	Vinyl chloride	Creech and Johnson, 1974; Waxweiler et al., 1976; Spirtas and Kaminski, 1978.

Table 9.4 (continued)

Site	Agent or Industrial Process	References
Lung, Bronchus	Arsenic (inorganic compounds)	Hill and Faning, 1948; Roth, 1958; Galy et al., 1963; Lee and Fraumeni, 1969; Ott et al., 1974; Milham and Strong, 1974; Kuratsune et al., 1974; Tokudome and Kuratsune, 1976; Rencher et al., 1977; Pinto et al., 1978; Axelson et al., 1978; Mabuchi et al., 1980.
	Asbestos	Merewether, 1949; Doll, 1955; Mancuso and Coulter, 1963; Selikoff et al., 1964; Jacob and Anspach, 1965; Lieben, 1966; Enterline and Kendrick, 1967; Selikoff et al., 1968; Knox et al., 1968; Newhouse, 1969; Tabershaw et al., 1970; Elmes and Simpson, 1971; Fletcher, 1972; Selikoff et al., 1972; Newhouse et al., 1972; Enterline et al., 1973; Selikoff et al., 1973; Edge, 1976; Martischnig et al., 1977; Peto et al., 1977; Robinson et al., 1979; McDonald et al, 1980; Selikoff et al., 1980.
	Bis (chloromethyl) ether	Figueroa et al., 1973; Lemen et al., 1976; DeFonso and Kelton, 1976; Pasternack et al., 1977.
	Chromium compounds	Machle and Gregorious, 1948; Baetjer, 1950a; Baetjer, 1950b; Mancuso and Hueper, 1951; Brinton et al., 1952; Bidstrup and Case, 1956; Enterline, 1974; Langard and Norseth, 1975; Royle, 1975; Michel-Briand and Simonin, 1977; Davies, 1978; Hayes et al., 1979; Dalager et al., 1980.

Source: D. Schottenfeld and J. Fraumeni, *Cancer Epidemiology and Prevention* (New York: W. B. Saunders, 1982).
*Note: Although this information dates to a 1982 source, the facts are still current in 1994.

Table 9.5
Industrial Materials for Which
Epidemiologic Studies Suggest Carcinogenicity*

Material	Site(s)	References
Acrylonitrile	Lung	O'Berg, 1980.
Asbestos	Colon, Rectum	Selikoff et al., 1973.
	Esophagus	Selikoff et al., 1973.
	Larynx	Steil and McGill, 1973; Shetti-gara and Morgan, 1975.
	Stomach	Selikoff et al., 1973.
Beryllium	Lung	Mancuso, 1980; Wagoner et al., 1980.
Cadmium	Lung	Lemen et al., 1976.
	Prostate	Potts, 1965; Kipling and Water-house, Lemen et al., 1976.
Coke Oven	Kidney	Redmond et al., 1973.
Emissions	Prostate	Redmond et al., 1973.
Cutting Oils	Lung, Digestive organs	Waterhouse, 1972.
	Stomach, Large intestine	Decoufle, 1978.
	Stomach	Jarvholm et al., 1981.
Ethylene Oxide/	Blood (leukemia)	Hogstedt et al., 1979
Ethylene Dichloride	Stomach	Hogstedt et al., 1979
Lead	Lung	Cooper and Gaffey, 1975.
Polychlorinated Biphenyis	Skin (melanoma)	Bahn et al., 1976.
Vinyl Chloride	Brain	Waxweiler et al., 1976
	Lung	Waxweiler et al., 1976

Source: D. Schottenfeld and J. Fraumeni, *Cancer Epidemiology and Prevention* (New York: W. B. Saunders, 1982).
*Note: Although this information dates to a 1982 source, the facts are still current in 1994.

Table 9.6
Occupational Groups Associated with High Risks for Cancer, with No Specific Agents Identified*

Benzoyl Chloride Manufacture	Lung	Sakabe et al., 1976.
Chemists	Brain	Olin and Ahibom, 1980.
	Lymphatic and Hematopoietic Tissues	Li et al., 1969; Olin and Ahibom, 1980.
	Pancreas	Li et al., 1969.
Coal Miners	Stomach	Rockette, 1977.
Coke By-Product Plant Workers	Colon	Redmond et al., 1976.
	Pancreas	Redmond et al., 1976.
Foundry Workers	Lung	Turner and Grace, 1938; McLaughlin and Harding, 1956; Koskela et al., 1976; Gibson et al., 1977; Decoufle and Wood, 1979; Egan et al., 1979; Tola et al., 1979.
Leather Workers	Bladder	Henry et al., 1931; Versluys, 1949; Wynder et al., 1963; Cole et al., 1972; Decoufle, 1979
	Larynx	Decoufle, 1979.
	Mouth, Pharynx	Decoufle, 1979.
Metal Miners	Lung	Wagoner et al., 1963.
Oil Refinery/ Petrochemical Workers	Brain	Theriault and Goulet, 1979; Alexander et al., 1980.
	Brain, Leukemia, Multiple Myeloma, Stomach	Thomas et al., 1980.
	Esophagus, Lung, Stomach	Hains et al., 1979.
Painters	Blood (leukemia)	Viadana and Bross, 1972.

Table 9.6 (continued)

Printing Workers	Lung	Moss et al., 1972; Greenberg, 1972.
	Mouth, Pharynx	Lloyd et al., 1977.
Rubber Industry Work Areas	Bladder	Monson and Nakano, 1976; McMichael et al., 1976; Monson and Fine, 1978.
	Blood (leukemia)	Monson and Nakano, 1976; McMichael et al., 1976; Andjelkovich et al., 1977; Monson and Fine, 1978.
	Brain	Monson and Nakano, 1976; Monson and Fine, 1978.
	Lung	Monson and Nakano, 1976; McMichael et al., 1976; Fox and Collier, 1976; Andjelkovich et al., 1977; Monson and Fine, 1978.
	Prostate	McMichael et al., 1976; Andjelkovich et al., 1977.
	Stomach	Monson and Nakano, 1976; McMichael et al., 1976; Andjelkovich et al., 1977; Monson and Fine, 1978.
Textile Workers	Nasal Cavity and Sinuses	Acheson et al., 1972.
Woodworkers	Lymphatic Tissue (Hodgkin's disease)	Milham and Hesser, 1967; Petersen and Milham, 1974; Grufferman et al., 1976; Greene et al., 1978.

Source: D. Schottenfeld and J. Fraumeni, *Cancer Epidemiology and Prevention* (New York: W. B. Saunders, 1982).
*Note: Although this information dates to a 1982 source, the facts are still current in 1994.

10

Diet and Cancer

The proliferation of official dietary recommendations has encouraged the public to conclude that diet is a very important factor in the cause and prevention of cancer. A widely circulated set of estimates of the proportions of cancer deaths attributable to various factors gives the same impression. According to these estimates, shown in Table 10.1, diet is responsible for 35 percent of all cancer deaths, making it the single largest cause of cancer—more important even than tobacco.

These estimates are legitimate indeed; they are the work of two of the world's most eminent epidemiologists, but they can easily mislead nonscientists who may not realize that there are vast differences in the certainty of the various estimates and in their usefulness in cancer prevention.

But people need to acknowledge that this 35 percent estimate is exactly that: a ballpark figure. The actual total may be as low as 10 percent or as high as 70 percent. In addition, scientists do not yet know exactly what the key

Table 10.1
Proportions of Cancer Deaths
Attributed to Various Factors

Factor	Percent of All Cancer Deaths (Best Estimate)
Diet	35
Tobacco	30
Infection	10?
Reproductive and sexual behavior	7
Occupation	4
Geophysical factors	3
Alcohol	3
Pollution	2
Industrial products	1
Food additives	1
Medicines and medical procedures	1
Unknown	?

Source: R. Doll and R. Peto, "The Causes of Cancer: Quantitative Estimates of Avoidable Risks of Cancer in the United States Today," *Journal of the National Cancer Institute* 66 (1981): 1191–1308.

dietary factors are, or exactly what people should eat in order to minimize their risk of cancer. (In contrast, the 30 percent estimate for tobacco is reasonably firm.)

Scientific Studies of Diet and Cancer

Cancer researchers conduct several different types of epidemiological studies to identify possible cancer risks.

In *correlational* investigations, scientists compare groups of people with different rates of a disease to see whether they differ in a particular risk factor. For instance, researchers might investigate whether levels of fat intake in various countries are correlated with the rates of particular types of cancer in those countries. Studies of this type are useful for generating new ideas, but their findings must be interpreted with caution. It is difficult to determine whether those in whom the disease develops are typical or atypical members of their particular group. It is also important to recognize that a correlation may not necessarily reflect a cause-and-effect relationship. For example, as societies develop, markets for consumer goods such as cigarettes and toilet paper increase. Because of this, there is a correlation between death from lung cancer and per capita toilet paper use, although few would seriously propose a cause-effect link.

Case-control and *cohort* studies focus on individuals rather than population groups. In case-control studies, individuals who have the disease under investigation are compared with otherwise similar individuals who do not have the disease, to see how they may differ. These studies are retrospective at the time of the investigation, the cases are already ill, and the focus is on past dietary habits (and other factors) that may have influenced their current state of health.

In cohort studies, researchers recruit groups of people who do not have the disease under investigation and investigate various aspects of their health and lifestyles. They then observe these subjects over a period of time. At the end of the follow-up period, subjects who develop the disease are compared with those who do not. Cohort studies are prospective, meaning that information about the subjects is collected before any of them become ill.

Although both of these study designs have potential

limitations, cohort studies are generally less susceptible to bias because the data are collected before the disease occurs. However, cohort studies are much more difficult and expensive than case-control studies, they require much larger numbers of subjects, and they take many years to complete. Most studies of diet and cancer are of the case-control type. In the past few years, however, findings from several large cohort studies have become available, and they have made important contributions to scientific understanding of the roles of various dietary factors.

One other important type of study is the *intervention* trial, in which the investigator randomly assigns the subjects to two groups, which are either exposed or not exposed to the factor under investigation. Studies of this type are ideal for establishing true cause-and-effect relationships, but they are extremely difficult to conduct when the factors of interest are complex, as diet is, or when the disease takes many years to develop, as cancer does. A few long-term intervention studies involving relatively simple diet modifications (such as taking or not taking a vitamin supplement) are currently in progress, and results will become available within the next decade.

This chapter on diet and cancer is divided into three parts: what people think causes cancer, what really does cause cancer, and dietary advice to prevent cancer.

What Dietary Factors Are Thought to Cause Cancer?

From cured and pickled meats to saccharin, food additives and chemicals used by the food industry such as Alar and EDB—what is a proven cause of cancer in humans?

CURED, SMOKED, AND PICKLED FOODS

In the early 1980s, the National Research Council recommended that people minimize intake of foods preserved by saltcuring, saltpickling, or smoking. By 1989, the National Research Council no longer included this advice in their dietary guidelines.

In some parts of the world where heavily smoked, salted, and/or pickled foods are consumed on a daily basis as major dietary items, the death rates from cancers of the esophagus and stomach are very high. Carcinogens are known to be present in foods preserved in these traditional ways, and they are believed to contribute to the high risks of stomach and esophageal cancers.

In the United States, however, esophageal cancer is very rare, and the death rate from stomach cancer has been declining steadily for more than half a century. During the same time period, consumption of processed (cured/smoked) meat in the United States has increased substantially. There is no epidemiological evidence linking increased consumption of processed meats in the United States with increased risks of any types of cancer.

Why is the relationship between cured/smoked foods and cancer different in the United States than in some other countries? The main reason seems to be differences in the food products themselves. The cured or smoked foods most commonly consumed in the United States, such as frankfurters, ham, and bacon, are very different from the foods that have been linked with increased cancer risks in countries such as China, Japan, and Iceland. Most of the cured, smoked, or salted foods sold in the United States have received only mild treatments that give them their characteristic flavor and appearance; few products are treated to the extent needed to render them stable without refrigeration. In other countries, such foods are significantly more heavily cured, smoked or salted.

In 1994, the evidence for the carcinogenicity of cured, pickled or salted foods in the United States is definitely waning.

FOOD "CHEMICALS" AND CANCER

A plethora of myths surround the issue of food additives and cancer. Many Americans stand ready to accuse food colors, stabilizers and flavorants of causing widespread cancer.

None of the expert groups that have issued dietary recommendations for cancer prevention, however, has advised Americans to avoid foods containing artificial additives, preservatives, pesticide residues, or other "chemicals." This consensus is based on the extensive research failing to find any evidence linking added chemicals in the U.S. food supply with increased risks of any type of cancer.

Let's look at a few of these.

Red Dye No. 2. It seems that food dyes are under intense scrutiny as a cause of human cancer. Red Dye No. 2 (also called amaranth), for example, was widely used in soft drinks, ice cream, baked goods, candy and other foods. Although this dye was used extensively in the United States since the turn of the century without any reported risk to human health, it was called into question in 1972 after Russian scientists suggested it might cause cancer in animals. Although no one really knew how reliable the Russian studies were (or even the purity of the dye used in their testing), damaging doubts had been raised. Despite the fact that one positive test in this country was refuted by dozens of negative tests, Red No. 2 was banned in 1976—the prevailing fear of cancer won out.

Red No. 3 came under similar scrutiny in 1990 after male rats fed very high doses developed tumors. The FDA soon called for a partial ban of this dye, which, oddly enough, only affected about 20 percent of its use. The ban doesn't affect the majority of approved uses, such as in fruit juices, gelatin desserts and fruit-cocktail cherries. This was a classic example of cancer hysteria prompting an illogical action.

Alar. There probably isn't an American who doesn't remember the scare with apples that hit the airwaves in 1989. Alar, an apple growth regulator with the chemical name daminozide used to help apples stay on trees longer to ripen (thus increasing yield), was indicted as a cause of human cancer. The "news" hit the airwaves in a big way, thanks to a carefully orchestrated media extravaganza that didn't leave one network or major newspaper out of the picture.

Contrary to what you read and heard everywhere about Alar, there simply was no proof that it caused human cancer. Shocking, isn't it, considering how the news was hammered into all of us? The U.S. Environmental Protection Agency estimates that the doses used in (questionable) animal studies were over one-half million times normal human ingestion. And it should be emphasized that the one study used by alarmists was never published in a reputable journal, being called under serious question because of its inadequacies.

Most telling are the comments of a cancer expert from the National Cancer Institute, Richard Adamson, M.D., who said of Alar: "The risk of eating an apple treated with Alar is less than the risk of eating a peanut butter sandwich or a well done hamburger."

Unfortunately, Alar was banned, devastating the apple industry and also frightening people unnecessarily. The losses to the apple industry were estimated at $250 million; and apple growers have forever lost a product that was extremely useful to their industry.

Saccharin. Saccharin became a cause célèbre in March 1977, when the FDA announced its intention to ban the sweetener in response to a Canadian study of saccharin and bladder cancer in rats. Acting in response to a massive public mandate, Congress passed the Saccharin Study and Labeling Act before the proposed ban could go into effect. This act imposed a moratorium on the FDA action. Later Congressional actions have extended that moratorium and kept saccharin on the market.

Does this mean that the American public is being unnecessarily exposed to a cancer hazard? Definitely not. The totality of the evidence gathered from the numerous animal and human studies of saccharin does not confirm that there is any risk to the human population from the use of normal amounts of it. Saccharin has been studied so extensively that we can answer all of the questions about the relative hazards of carcinogens that were posed in the previous section. Let's look at those answers.

How potent a carcinogen is saccharin? It's the *weakest* carcinogen ever discovered through animal testing. Every other confirmed carcinogen you've ever heard of, including all of the naturally occurring food carcinogens discussed earlier in this chapter, is more potent than saccharin.

Does it show signs of being particularly dangerous? No,

in fact the evidence suggests that its hazards are very limited. It causes tumors only in male rats, not in any other type of animal studied. It causes tumors only when administered for a lifetime, starting at conception or birth (even weaning to death is not a long enough period to cause tumor development). The tumors occur in one body organ only, the bladder. Bladder tumors also occur spontaneously in rats. The bladder tumors produced by saccharin do not kill the rats.

What about dose/response relationships? Saccharin is one of the few substances for which an adequate dose/response study has been performed. That study showed that the tumor rate is definitely not proportional to the dose of saccharin administered. Instead, the incidence of tumors declines very sharply with a decrease in dose.

How do levels of human exposure compare to doses that have produced cancer in animals? Mathematical models have been used to estimate the hypothetical increased risk of bladder cancer that could be caused by exposure to saccharin at ordinary human exposure levels. Based on the dose/response study data, the modes indicated that exposure to saccharin at normal dietary levels for a lifetime would increase the chance of developing bladder cancer by considerably less than one in a million.

Is there human evidence? Yes, an unusually large amount of it, and it does not indicate a hazard. This evidence includes an extremely large case-control study conducted by the National Cancer Institute. More than 9,000 people were studied, and no association was found between artificial sweetener use and bladder cancer in the overall groups of men, women, or both sexes combined.

The human evidence also includes studies of people with

unusually high saccharin exposures, namely, diabetics. Presumably, if saccharin posed a cancer risk, these heavy users would have a greater risk than those consuming more moderate amounts. Studies of diabetics have reported no association between saccharin use and the occurrence of bladder cancer. Indeed, saccharin is an excellent example of the sort of animal carcinogen that is not worth worrying about.

So why was there so much fuss about saccharin? Why was it nearly banned? Because saccharin is a food additive, and the law imposes stricter standards on this class of food ingredient than on other food constituents. Food constituents are currently regulated on the basis of how they find their way into food, not on the basis of how much of a hazard they may pose. This policy is contrary to current scientific evidence. In fact, if we applied the food additive standards to everything we eat, we would starve, because virtually all natural foods would flunk the tests for one reason or another.

Ethylene Dibromide (EDB) is a pesticide, which, until 1984, had four important agricultural uses. It was used as a pre-plant fumigant to control nematodes in soil, particularly in the citrus industry. It was used for the bulk fumigation of stored grains, eliminating prolific beetles, weevils, and other insects. EDB was used to kill insects in the milling machinery used to grind grain into flour. It was also used to fumigate the relatively small amount of fruit shipped from one fruit-growing region to another to prevent the spread of fruit flies.

Virtually all uses of EDB were ended by a ban in 1984. The ban was accompanied by a massive public panic over even small traces of EDB residues in foods. Did the ban make sense? Was the panic justified? Let's look again at the same sorts of questions that we posed for saccharin.

How potent a carcinogen is EDB? On the full range of carcinogenic potencies for chemicals, it is right in the middle. If one looked only at pesticides, EDB would be one of the most potent carcinogens. It must be remembered, however, that the term "potency" refers merely to the amount of a chemical needed to produce cancer in animals. The degree of hazard also depends on how much of the chemical people are exposed to, as will be discussed below.

Does EDB show signs of being a particularly dangerous carcinogen? To some degree, yes. Three long-term, high-dose cancer studies on EDB have been carried out using two routes of administration in both sexes of two species of test animals, and EDB unequivocally increased the rate of cancer in all of them. Tumors started appearing in the animals at an early age. EDB represents greater potential hazard than saccharin.

Do we have dose/response data? As is the case with most substances, the answer, unfortunately, is no. How do the levels of human exposure compare to the levels that have caused cancer in animals? Human exposure levels are much, much lower. It was confusion over the contrasting facets of the EDB problem—that consumers were exposed to *tiny* amounts of a *potent* carcinogen—that generated much of the public misunderstanding.

The Environmental Protection Agency (EPA) estimated that the average pre-ban consumer intake of EDB was in the range of five to ten micrograms per person per day. This is a very small amount. For comparison, we typically ingest 140,000 micrograms of pepper per day. Ten micrograms per person per day of EDB is less than a quarter-millionth as much, on a proportional body weight basis, as the rats were given in the cancer tests. To put it another way, you would have to eat 250,000 times as much food as you normally do in order to equal the cancer-producing dose fed to the laboratory animals.

The hypothetical cancer risk from these extremely small amounts of EDB vanishes into insignificance against the background of other, natural carcinogens in food. For instance, pepper was mentioned earlier, and it is known to contain carcinogens. At the typical daily doses of ingestion, pepper poses ten to one hundred times the carcinogenic risk of EDB in food. And nobody is talking about banning pepper, quite correctly, since even this risk is too small for serious concern.

Aflatoxin provides another useful comparison. As discussed below, it is a real problem if present in large amounts. But at the tiny levels permitted by the FDA, it is generally agreed not to pose a significant hazard. Yet if you calculate out the carcinogenic potencies of aflatoxin and EDB and examine the maximum permitted residue levels for the two substances, you will find that the government permits consumers to be exposed to 667 times the carcinogenic hazard from aflatoxin as from EDB. And again, this does not pose a risk to public health.

What about human evidence on EDB? Fortunately, we have some, and it comes from studies of workers occupationally exposed to much larger amounts of EDB than the general public would ever have encountered. Such studies are particularly likely to detect adverse effects, if such effects exist.

The workers studied had been exposed to doses some five to ten thousand times higher than consumers for periods up to sixteen years or more. The incidence of cancer among them was not significantly different from that expected in an unexposed population. Of course, since the groups of workers were relatively small, we cannot say that the studies prove that EDB does not cause cancer. But the fact that no increase in cancer was seen even at these extremely high doses tells us that the risk to consumers at the doses they were exposed to before the ban is at most exceedingly small.

What about substitutes for EDB? This is the most unfortunate part of the EDB problem, because EDB has now been replaced by other fumigants which are less satisfactory, both in terms of function and health effects. The major substitutes for EDB are methyl bromide and phosphine. Neither can be used for spot fumigation, an important pre-ban use of EDB. Methyl bromide is a proven carcinogen. Phosphine has never been adequately tested for carcinogenicity. Both substances are much more hazardous to the workers who must use them than EDB was. Both are much more poisonous than EDB, and methyl bromide has the additional hazard of being odorless at concentrations high enough to be toxic, so workers are not warned of leaks by any telltale odor. Phosphine has the additional hazard of being highly flammable.

In sum, EDB's replacements offer little, if any, improvement over EDB with regard to their intrinsic carcinogenicity, and they have substantial safety disadvantages for workers.

So were the government's actions against EDB justified? In part, yes. It wasn't until February 1984 that tolerance levels were set for EDB in foods. EDB is a potent carcinogen that deserves to be taken seriously. Clearly, this important action was long overdue. However, the rest of the government actions—the ban on most uses of EDB—do not appear to have been justified. The hazard eliminated was at most extremely small. In addition, because of the lack of fully adequate substitutes the overall impact of the EDB ban on health and safety was negative. The public panic over EDB was certainly unwarranted. As one prominent scientist pointed out, all of the people who returned EDB-contaminated foods to the market were in far greater danger of being killed in an auto accident during that extra trip to the store than they could possibly have been from the EDB residues in the foods. But in this case as in many others, the public was not given the complete information needed to evaluate the hazard properly. Instead, both government and the press (notably the TV network which showed a skull and crossbones on the screen every time the EDB issue was discussed on its news broadcasts) seemed to promote public fears rather than really informing people.

Coffee and tea. Two important sources of "chemicals" in the U.S. diet are coffee and tea, both of which contain a wide variety of chemical substances. However, there is no convincing evidence linking either coffee or tea with increased cancer risks in humans. In some epidemiological studies, increased intake of coffee has been associated with higher risks of bladder cancer, but experts suspect that this may reflect some kind of bias rather than a cause-and-effect relationship. Coffee consumption is associated with an increased risk of fibrocystic breast disease but not with breast cancer.

What Constituents of Food Really Cause Cancer?

CONTAMINATING MICROORGANISMS

In some non-Western societies, certain "chemicals" in food have been linked with increased cancer risks. For example, certain parts of China have unusually high rates of naso-pharyngeal, esophageal, and stomach cancers, which have been linked to the heavy consumption of certain traditionally preserved (salted or fermented) foods. These foods may contain carcinogenic chemicals produced by the preservation process or by the actions of contaminating microorganisms. In some parts of Asia and Africa, high rates of liver cancer may be related to the consumption of foods contaminated with aflatoxin or other chemical substances produced by molds. These toxins can form in grains, peanuts, or other foods stored under less-than-optimal conditions, particularly in warm, moist climates.

In the United States, on the other hand, mold contamination is limited by good storage practices and foods are preserved primarily by refrigeration, freezing, and canning, rather than by traditional methods of fermentation. Exposure to harmful contaminants is minimal and the associated cancer risk infinitesimally small.

NATURAL CARCINOGENS

Probably one of the most underappreciated facts about the cancer-causing potential of the American diet has to do with carcinogens found naturally—meaning nature put them there—in food. The quantity of natural mutagens and carcinogens in food is believed to be greater, by several orders of magnitude, than the quantity of man-made mutagens and carcinogens.

Cinnamon and black pepper contain the natural carcinogen safrole. Baked potatoes have arsenic (and other potential mutagens) and mushrooms hydrazines. Mustard, horseradish, and cabbage sport a little allyl isothiocyanate. Despite the plethora of naturally occurring carcinogenic substances in food, there is little evidence linking any of these natural carcinogens with increased cancer risks in humans.

Indeed, there is no need to eliminate such foods from your diet. It might even be counterproductive to do so, since many of the foods that contain carcinogens also contain anti-carcinogens, and we do not know which substances are more important.

This also points to two extremely important points. First is a major presumption we should forthrightly reject: that "natural" is safe and "man-made" suspect. It also brings up the quintessential adage "Only the dose makes the poison." Nearly four tons of turkey would be needed to deliver a toxic dose of malonaldehyde—all at one sitting. A perspective sorely lacking in this country is that we readily accept much higher levels of naturally occurring *proven* carcinogens, yet quickly reject much, much smaller levels of synthetic substances never shown to cause cancer.

Can Diet Prevent Cancer?

FRUITS, VEGETABLES, AND CANCER

As recently as the mid-1980s, vegetables and fruits merited only a brief mention. At that time, the evidence that these foods might protect against cancer was not very strong. In the few short intervening years, the situation—and resultant advice—has changed considerably.

Today an impressive body of scientific evidence links high intakes of fruits and vegetables with decreased risks of a wide variety of cancers. Almost two hundred epidemiological studies have examined the effects of fruits and vegetables, and the vast majority have found that people who eat more fruits and vegetables have lower cancer risks. The evidence is particularly strong for cancers of the lung, larynx, oral cavity, pharynx, and esophagus, and there is also substantial evidence of protective effects against cancers of the pancreas, stomach, colon, rectum, bladder, breast, cervix, ovary, and endometrium. In fact, the only major site for which the epidemiological evidence is inconclusive is the prostate.

The association between fruit and vegetable intake and cancer risk is large enough to be of practical importance. For most cancer sites, people with low intakes of these foods have about twice the risk of cancer seen in those with high intakes.

It has been argued that the apparent protective effect of fruits and vegetables might actually be due to the substitution of these foods for other foods associated with increased risk, such as meat or fat. However, enough data have accumulated now to rule out this possibility. Fruits and vegetables have been linked with decreased cancer risks in a wide variety of populations from around the world, including many groups that do not have the same pattern of correlated dietary habits found in the United States. For example, in developing countries, people who don't eat fruits and vegetables compensate by eating more of their staple grain foods, not more meat and fat, yet fruits and vegetables are protective in those populations just as they are in the United States.

THE ROLE OF ANTIOXIDANT VITAMINS

There is a strong biological rationale for a protective effect of fruits and vegetables. These foods are the principal dietary sources of vitamin C and carotenoids,* and they are also a major source of vitamin E. All three of these nutrients are antioxidants, meaning that they can block or repair damage caused by free radicals and other highly reactive chemical entities produced by oxidation. Free radicals and other reactive oxygen species are formed as byproducts of normal metabolism or in response to external stressors such as tobacco smoke.

Other components of fruits and vegetables, including the B vitamin folic acid and certain nonnutritive substances such as indoles, may also contribute to cancer prevention; their roles and biochemical effects are not well understood. Some authorities strongly recommend the consumption of cruciferous (cabbage family) vegetables, such as broccoli and cauliflower, because they are rich in nonnutritive substances that may act as cancer inhibitors. However, the evidence for benefits attributable to this specific subgroup of vegetables is not very strong.

---

*Carotenoids are a group of red, orange, and yellow pigments found in plants. They are responsible for the colors of many vegetables and a few fruits, including carrots, sweet potatoes, tomatoes, corn, and cantaloupe. Dark green vegetables, such as spinach and broccoli, also contain carotenoids, but in these foods the characteristic colors of the carotenoid pigments are masked by the green color of chlorophyll. Some carotenoids can be converted to vitamin A in the body; others cannot. However, vitamin A activity does not appear to be important in cancer prevention.

It may be many years before scientists fully understand the relative importance of various components of fruits and vegetables and the exact actions of each of these substances. However, it is not necessary to wait for a full understanding of the biochemistry before making sensible public health recommendations.

All Americans should include at least five servings of fruits and vegetables in their daily diets. In most epidemiological studies, this level of consumption has been associated with substantial reductions in cancer risk. It is a good idea to frequently choose fruits and vegetables that are rich in carotenoids or vitamin C. Because the evidence for a protective effect of cruciferous vegetables is still weak, it may not be necessary to push these vegetables. Table 10.2 lists some of the best fruit and vegetable choices and gives information on how to prepare these foods in ways that preserve their vitamin C content.

The recommended level of fruit and vegetable consumption may have other health benefits in addition to its association with cancer prevention, and it is unlikely to cause any adverse health effects.

Some epidemiological evidence links fruits and vegetables, and the antioxidants that they contain, with decreased risk of cataracts. Some fruits and vegetables provide fiber, which is generally considered desirable for good health. Fruits, as consumed, are relatively low in fat and calories and thus may be a desirable substitute for higher fat, higher calorie foods. (This may help maintain a lean body weight, which is very critical to good health.) Vegetables are also low in fat and calories if they are cooked without added fat and served plain. However, in practice, people often add fat to vegetables either in cooking or at the table (in the

Table 10.2
For Good Nutrition, Experts Recommend That Everyone Should Have at Least 3 Servings of Vegetables and at Least 2 Servings of Fruit Every Day

What Counts as One Serving?

1 cup of raw leafy green vegetables
½ cup of other raw or cooked vegetables
1 piece of fruit
1 wedge of melon
¾ cup of juice
½ cup of canned fruit
¼ cup of dried fruit

The Best Sources of Beta-Carotene and other Carotenoids

orange-yellow vegetables (carrots, sweet potatoes, winter squash)
dark-green leafy vegetables (spinach, kale, collards)
broccoli
orange-yellow non-citrus fruits (canteloupe, apricots)

The Best Sources of Vitamin C

citrus fruits (oranges, grapefruit, tangerines)
strawberries
certain vegetables (peppers, tomatoes, cabbage, broccoli, cauliflower)

To Preserve the Vitamin C Content of Foods

Eat some fruits and vegetables raw, since cooking decreases vitamin C levels
Cook vegetables in minimal amounts of water and only until they reach the crisp-tender stage.

form of butter, margarine, cooking fats, sauces, mayonnaise, or salad dressing). This increases the fat and calorie content of the vegetables but does not negate their other desirable characteristics.

CURRENT CONSUMPTION LEVELS

The recommendation to eat five servings of fruits and vegetables daily may not appear to be a startling change; after all, the Basic Four Food Groups plan that was in use for many decades called for four daily servings of these foods. However, while the new recommendation is not dramatically different from previous advice, it is very different from what Americans actually eat. For example, one major survey of a representative sample of the U.S. population showed that:

- 41 percent of the people surveyed had no fruit or fruit juice on the survey day.

- 17 percent had no vegetables on the survey day.

- Only 28 percent consumed a fruit or vegetable rich in vitamin C.

- Only 21 percent consumed a fruit or vegetable rich in carotenoids.

- Only 27 percent had the recommended three servings of vegetables.

- Only 30 percent had the recommended two servings of fruits.

- A mere 10 percent had three servings of vegetables and two servings of fruits on the survey day.

Clearly, there is plenty of room for improvement.

WHAT ABOUT VITAMIN SUPPLEMENTS?

Because fruits and vegetables have been linked with reduced cancer risks—explained most likely by their antioxidant vitamins—it is reasonable to ask whether Americans should be advised to take supplements of these nutrients. In 1994, the answer is probably "no."

The evidence for a cancer-protective effect of individual antioxidant vitamins is substantial, but it is not as extensive or convincing as the evidence for fruits and vegetables. Foods are chemically complex mixtures, and it is very difficult to disentangle the effects of specific components. Substances in fruits and vegetables other than the three antioxidant vitamins may prove to be very important in cancer prevention, and a variety of other carotenoids may prove to be at least as important as beta-carotene, the one carotenoid usually included in supplements. For these reasons, individuals who choose to take supplements instead of eating fruits and vegetables might end up with less effective health protection.

There is some reason for concern about the safety of antioxidant supplementation. Although the scientific evidence indicates that vitamin C, vitamin E, and beta-carotene are of low toxicity, even when consumed in doses far beyond those normally obtained from food, a few scientific findings suggest that consumption of large doses of these vitamins might not be safe for all subgroups of the population (especially people taking anti-coagulants and other medications.)

For example, in an experiment in baboons, beta-carotene supplementation worsened the liver damage caused by large doses of alcohol. Whether this finding can be extrapolated to human alcohol abusers is uncertain. Also, there have been some indications that large doses of beta-carotene might interfere with uptake of vitamin E in the intestine, and vice versa. Whether this effect is of any practical significance is unclear.

There is also legitimate reason for concern about the likelihood that people might take supplements inappropriately. Although the antioxidant vitamins are reasonably nontoxic, many other vitamins and minerals are not. They can cause serious harm if consumed in excessive doses. An individual who chose to increase his intake of antioxidants by taking several multivitamin tablets daily instead of one could be in serious trouble. Confusion about betacarotene and vitamin A is also a problem. Beta-carotene, which is a precursor of vitamin A and a strong antioxidant, is relatively nontoxic (although it can cause a reversible yellow discoloration of the skin if consumed in very large amounts). Vitamin A itself is not an antioxidant and is both toxic and teratogenic (capable of causing birth defects) if consumed in large doses.

Several intervention studies of the antioxidant vitamins are in progress, and others are planned. In these studies, large numbers of volunteers have been randomly assigned to take either a supplement or an inactive placebo on a regular basis for a period of years. Results of these intervention trials should become available within the next decade. At that time, it may be possible to make a definitive recommendation for or against the use of antioxidant supplements. By then, it is also likely that the small number of lingering concerns about the safety of the antioxidant vitamins will have been resolved by additional scientific research.

A PERSPECTIVE ON VITAMIN SUPPLEMENTS

Nutrition educators traditionally taught the public that the only function of vitamins was to prevent vitamin deficiency diseases. Intakes of vitamins at levels above the Recommended Dietary Allowances (RDA) were actively discouraged. Claims that vitamin doses above the RDA might have special health benefits were dismissed as scientifically unsound.

Recent findings, particularly those involving the antioxidant vitamins, have led nutrition scientists to reexamine these views. Sound scientific research, conducted in leading institutions, is beginning to show that some vitamins may indeed have functions beyond the prevention of deficiency. Of course, this does not mean that all of the claims that have ever been made about the benefits of vitamins are true. Most of those claims were unfounded and they remain unfounded. Health professionals and nutrition educators must face the challenging task of helping the public distinguish legitimate scientific facts about above RDA doses of vitamins from the continuing outpouring of vitamin folklore and quackery.

DIETARY FIBER AND CANCER

The idea that increased consumption of dietary fiber may reduce the risk of cancer has become part of the conventional nutrition wisdom in the U.S. Yet there is a lack of good scientific evidence to support this claim.

Researchers find dietary fiber difficult to study because it is not one substance but many, and different types of fiber can have different effects in the body. Also, people don't consume fiber in isolation; it occurs as a component of grain products, vegetables, and fruits that also contain many other components, some of which may influence cancer risk. For these reasons, the results of studies of dietary fiber have been complex and confusing.

Official recommendations often state that fiber may help to prevent "some" types of cancer. In fact, the "some" refers only to two closely related cancer sites—the colon and rectum. There has never been any substantial scientific evidence linking fiber intake to decreased risk of cancer at any other body site in humans.

The epidemiological evidence on dietary fiber and cancers of the colon and rectum is inconsistent. Correlational studies have generally shown that groups who eat more fiber in general or more grain foods have lower colon cancer rates. In these studies, vegetables and fruits and the fibers that they contain seemed to have little or no effect. In case-control studies, on the other hand, protective effects have generally been associated only with vegetable fiber intake, while cereal fibers have often shown no effect or have been associated with increases in colon cancer risk. Only a few cohort studies have been completed, and none has shown a strong effect of fiber.

Like the epidemiological findings, the results of animal experiments have been inconsistent. In fact, under certain experimental conditions, some types of fiber actually increased colon cancer rates in experimental animals.

Nearly ten years ago, one could describe the scientific evidence on fiber and colon cancer as "exceptionally equivocal and inconsistent." That conclusion remains valid in

1994—there simply is insufficient evidence to conclude that fiber will lower cancer risk.*

Dietary Fat, Calories and Cancer

Of all the dietary factors under investigation, dietary fat intake has received the greatest emphasis both in research studies and in advice given to the public for cancer prevention. Yet despite extensive investigation, the scientific evidence on dietary fat and cancer is far from conclusive.

COLON CANCER

The evidence that dietary fat may cause cancer is strongest for colon cancer. Animal experiments have suggested plausible mechanisms by which fat might influence the development of cancer at this site. Correlational studies have found strong associations between the amount of fat consumed in various countries and the rates of colon cancer in those countries. Many case-control studies have been completed, and most have linked higher total fat intakes with higher risks of colon cancer, although several studies have not found such an association. A very large cohort study involving more than 80,000 female American nurses found higher rates of colon cancer in women with higher intakes of animal fat.

Some uncertainties remain, however. One major problem in the interpretation of these studies is that diets high in fat are usually high in calories as well, and it may be that

---

*People do need a reasonable dietary fiber for other health reasons, such as to ensure regularity.

total energy (calorie) intake, rather than fat specifically, is the key factor. In experimental animals, calories are more important than fat; test animals raised on a high-calorie, low-fat diet have higher cancer rates than those raised on a low-calorie, high-fat diet. Whether the same is true in humans is uncertain. Because of the high correlation between fat intake and calorie intake in human populations, epidemiological studies have not been able to make a clear distinction between the two factors.

BREAST CANCER

The evidence linking dietary fat to breast cancer is less convincing than that for colon cancer. The findings from case-control studies have been less consistent than those for colon cancer, and any effects noted have usually been weak. A Canadian cohort study showed some evidence of a positive association between dietary fat intake and breast cancer risk, but three other cohort studies (the U.S. Nurses' Study, a smaller study of a representative sample of the U.S. population, and a large study of postmenopausal women in the Netherlands) found no association.

As is the case for colon cancer, it is possible that total caloric intake may be more important than fat intake in determining breast cancer risk. There is also some reason to suspect that dietary factors might exert effects only in the early stages of life. If this is true, dietary changes later in life would not be worthwhile. It has also been suggested that only a drastic reduction in fat intake would be sufficient to cause a substantial decrease in the incidence of breast cancer. This argument may be valid, but its practical relevance is questionable, since an extreme reduction in dietary fat is unlikely to be achievable or acceptable in Western societies.

Some scientists still hope that it may be possible to decrease the incidence of breast cancer by reducing dietary fat intake.

PROSTATE CANCER

The evidence on dietary fat and prostate cancer is much less extensive than that for cancers of the breast and colon. Links between fat intake and prostate cancer risk have been made from some case-control studies, but sometimes only in certain age groups or for specific fat sources. Cohort studies have had inconsistent results. The ways in which fat might influence prostate cancer risk are poorly understood because there is no good animal model of this disease. Another complicating factor affecting all studies of prostate cancer is the high rate of latent disease. The ways in which men with latent prostate cancer may differ from those with clinically apparent, life-threatening disease are not well understood. In summary, the evidence on dietary fat intake and prostate cancer is inconclusive.

OTHER CANCER SITES

Animal experiments indicate that high dietary fat intake may increase the risk of pancreatic cancer. Whether this finding can be extrapolated to humans is unknown. Human pancreatic cancer is rapidly fatal; few patients live long enough to be interviewed by epidemiological researchers. Because investigation of this disease is so difficult, little is known about its risk factors.

Since cancers of the ovary and endometrium (lining of the uterus) are influenced by hormonal factors, which, in turn, can be influenced by diet, it is reasonable to propose that dietary fat intake might be associated with these cancers. However, only a very small number of studies of dietary factors and endometrial or ovarian cancer have been completed, and their findings are inconclusive.

RECOMMENDATIONS ON DIETARY FAT INTAKE

Virtually all health authorities have called for decreases in total fat intake, usually to 30 percent of total calories. Although fat's association with cancer has not been proven definitively, there are other health reasons to heed this lean advice. Consuming more than 30 percent of your diet as fat generally means you are skimping on some other healthy component of your diet—and studies have shown that these components are generally complex carbohydrates found in fruits, vegetables, and grains.

In addition, people who eat excess fat calories generally eat too many total calories, which often pushes them over the edge into obesity—which we know has proven detrimental effects on health. Finally, there is a growing body of evidence that excess fat calories lead to weight gain faster than do protein or carbohydrate calories.

OBESITY

There is some epidemiologic evidence supporting an association between excess weight and cancer. A large American Cancer Society study showed that cancer death rates increased progressively with increasing degrees of overweight in both men and women. Obesity has been linked to increased risks of endometrial cancer and postmenopausal breast cancer in women.

The current evidence linking obesity to cancer, if considered alone, would be insufficient to justify any recommendations to the public. However, obesity, as we mentioned above, is associated with several other diseases, including diabetes, high blood pressure, and coronary heart disease, and is clearly detrimental to health. All Americans should make an effort to maintain a healthful body weight through appropriate eating and exercise habits.

Diet and Cancer: Conclusions

This chapter has examined the multifaceted subject of diet and cancer, looking first at what frightens people most— food additives and other synthetic chemicals that end up in the food supply. Our second look was at something that is, at least theoretically, a more significant risk—natural carcinogens—but is essentially dismissed as people fret misguidedly over the former.

Finally, we've left you with some practical advice about a diet that will promote good health, and hopefully long life and may—we stress may—reduce your risk of cancer. Namely, there is growing evidence that some property of fruits and vegetables, most likely the natural antioxidants they contain, may reduce cancer risk. The other payoff in cancer prevention may be in achieving and maintaining a healthy body weight. As we already know the other benefits of doing so, we needn't wait.

We have one of the healthiest, and definitely one of the

most abundant supplies of food in the world. Instead of worrying about an artificial chemical that makes healthy, safe food available to us more readily—and with no discernible risk—we should be intent on trying to eat a healthy diet to achieve that lean body weight. The payoff is cancer prevention. Fretting over this or that chemical or food additive simply is not justifiable.

Finally, individuals who are setting their own health priorities should realize that the single most important step that people can take right now to reduce their risk of cancer is to abstain from using tobacco in any form. It is also important to emphasize that there is no known dietary change that will offset the harmful effects of cigarette smoking. People who believe that they can safely continue to smoke as long as they adhere to the latest dietary recommendations are deluding themselves.

Part Two

Myths and Secondary Prevention

11

Exploding Myths about
Purely Hypothetical Causes of Cancer

The preceding chapters have given you state-of-the-art information on the known (or in the case of diet, strongly suspected) causes of human cancer. As you read them, you may have been surprised by the omission of some well-publicized carcinogens from the list. Where were the cancer causes that you read about in the newspapers all the time—things like air and water pollutants, pesticides such as Alar and ethylene dibromide (EDB), food additives such as saccharin, the electricity from your alarm clock or cellular phone, and industrial chemicals in the environment such as polychlorinated biphenyls (PCBs)?

The reason that chapters on such substances were not included is that these agents have never been shown to pose a risk of human cancer. That's right; there's no evidence to convict them of causing cancer in humans. The others—the ones that make the headlines and have led to the common public perception that anything unpronounceable is likely to cause cancer—have *at most* shown signs of carcinogenicity only in animal tests or short-term assays. They are at most hypothetical cancer risks, yet they have received the bulk of the publicity. Worse yet, they have diverted our attention from the real and proven causes of cancer.

In order to make wise personal decisions about what we should do to reduce our individual risks of cancer and other serious health problems, we need to be able to distinguish real risks from those that are hypothetical. We have limited resources—we cannot devote our full attention to avoiding each and every hypothetical risk that finds its way to the six o'clock news. We must set priorities and focus our cancer prevention efforts on the things that matter— those with proven payoffs.

To help you in this admittedly difficult and confusing task, this chapter will critically review several of the best known cancer "scares," examine the kinds of evidence that have led certain man-made chemicals to be condemned in the headlines, and then evaluate the downside risks of the indiscriminate carcinogen busting that has dominated American regulatory philosophy for the past two decades. Let's look at some of these myths,* and then put them into perspective.

Is Dioxin the Most Toxic Substance Known to Man?

Over the past decade science has progressed at a remarkable pace. New advances and experimental results have changed

---

*We've already looked at some of these, such as EDB and saccharin, in chapter 10.

the prevailing theories regarding the impact of chemicals on human health. The new findings carry enough potential clout to slash multimillion dollar cleanup budgets across the country. The dioxin story at Times Beach illustrates this trend.

In 1982, more than 2,200 residents of Times Beach, Missouri, received emergency evacuation orders from top U.S. public health officials. Dioxin, they feared, posed an imminent threat to human health. Americans across the country, all too familiar with the dangerous reputation of dioxin, called for the removal of every last trace of dioxin at any cost. But ten years later, government officials and scientists, relying on new data and analysis, have stated that the evacuation was unnecessary. They had erred about dioxin's toxicity.

WHAT HAPPENED AT TIMES BEACH?

In the mid 1970s, thousands of gallons of waste oil were sprayed to reduce dust on a horse arena and unpaved roads in the Times Beach area. After horses and other animals in the immediate spraying area died, investigations pointed to dioxin, subsequently found to be a contaminant of the waste oil, as the culprit. The issue, however, lay dormant until December 1982 when flood waters spread the dioxin throughout the small town.

Federal officials were catapulted onto center stage by a critical, environmentally aware public who demanded an expedient remedy to assuage their fears. Soil levels measured 100 to 1,000 times what, at the time, was thought the safe limit of ingestion. A hasty evacuation was ordered, at a cost of $33 million dollars. The government's sense of urgency, coupled with research showing dioxin to be very carcinogenic in one laboratory animal species, was the stuff of which headline news is made. Dioxin was soon earmarked as environmental enemy number one, launched onto the front page and the first minutes of nearly every newscast.

A CLOSER LOOK AT THE FACTS

At the time of the evacuation, several facts suggested that, despite high soil dioxin levels, human health was not in jeopardy. Unequivocally, soil dioxin levels were high and had devastating effects on animals in the vicinity. But scientists knew that dioxin binds tightly to soil. This characteristic made human exposure very unlikely. It was highly improbable that humans were ingesting any of it.

In fact, there is no evidence that human health was or has been harmed as a result of high soil dioxin levels in Times Beach. There weren't even cases of chloracne, a reversible skin condition associated with significant dioxin exposure.

OLD FEARS REASSESSED

Dioxin was—and still is—notoriously referred to as "the most toxic substance known to man." But it is crucial to understand the roots of its heinous reputation.

Until the late 1980s, the potential human health effects of dioxin—and resultant public policies about the chemical— traced to a single 1978 rat study.

In that study, female rats which were fed excessively high doses of dioxin developed liver tumors. Two points are telling and are under intense scrutiny, though, as science has advanced. First, the liver tumors that developed in the rats were analyzed according to 1975 scientific criteria. Appropriate at the time, but not today, this evaluation suggested that dioxin was highly carcinogenic in that species. Second, these high dose experimental results were used to extrapolate the effects of low dose rat exposure. A second extrapolation, or projection, was then made to predict the health effects of low dose dioxin exposure in humans. In other words, scientists made two huge assumptions, thereby introducing enormous potential for error into their predictions.

It's not just that scientists extended the limits of a little knowledge to make predictions. Today, the same scientists seriously question how they stretched these facts. The projections were made according to standard protocol at the time, the linear dose model. This method assumes one can predict the consequences of low dose exposure from high dose exposures. The model assumes that some risk exists at every dose. That's like saying that because excessive calories cause weight gain, anything with calories causes obesity. Many scientists now recognize that this every-dose-has-a-risk philosophy is an inaccurate assumption.

Further, scientists have found a new, more accurate way to evaluate and classify the results of animal tests. Specifically, researchers have a more thorough understanding of how tumors develop when animals are fed extremely high levels of a chemical. When the original 1978 liver tumor samples were reevaluated with the new criteria developed from this clearer understanding, scientists were astounded to realize that tumors occurred only when the rats were fed doses large enough to kill cells. This caused the surviving cells to divide rapidly, in an effort to replace those cells that had not survived. Such hasty cell division can lead to mutations which can result in cancer.

Scientists discovered one additional crucial fact. For dioxin to even become poisonous, it must be given in a dose sufficiently large to activate certain body chemicals, called receptors. Below that critical dose, receptors simply don't function, and dioxin cannot possibly exert the toxic effect that leads to rapid cell division. There is absolutely no risk unless that critical dose is reached or exceeded.

Extensive human studies confirm that dioxin doesn't pose a significant human health threat. High-dose exposure can cause chloracne. However, there is no convincing evidence that dioxin causes any type of disease, adverse pregnancy outcome or premature mortality. There is a small, increased risk for cancer at very high exposures. Specifically, when blood levels of dioxin exceed 600 times the recognized background level, there is a very small (approximately one and one-half times) increased risk for all forms of cancer combined. Note, however, that such cancers occur only after a minimum of 20 years of exposure. To put this in perspective, consider that smokers are ten times more likely to get lung cancer than are non-smokers.

RETROSPECTIVE REGRETS AND A REEVALUATION

In an unprecedented action, EPA Administrator William K. Reilly set the regulatory works in action in April 1991. He ordered a reevaluation of the risks of dioxin exposure. He and other scientists have openly acknowledged the changing situation and have voiced their regrets about the Times Beach evacuation:

Given what we know about this chemical's toxicity and its effects on human health, it looks as though the evacuation was unnecessary. Times Beach was an over-reaction. It was based on the best scientific information we had at the time. It turns out we were in error. . . . The only thing I would have done differently, I would have said we may be wrong. If we're going to be wrong, we'll be wrong on the side of protecting human health. I don't think we ever said we may be wrong.

We're public health officials. When something is worse than we thought, we seem to be able to move very rapidly at gathering the data and making the decision to restrict its use. When something is not as bad as we thought it was, I think it's fair to bring that issue forward.

Vernon Houk, M.D.
Assistant Surgeon General and Director for the Center for Environmental Health and Injury Control at the Centers for Disease Control (the U.S. public health official who ordered the Times Beach evacuation)

I don't want to prejudge the issue, but we are seeing new information on dioxin that suggests a lower risk assessment for dioxin should be applied. . . . I know the stakes and that I'm unraveling something here. There isn't much precedent in the Federal establishment for pulling back from a judgment of toxicity. But we need to be prepared to adjust, to raise or lower standards, as new science becomes available.

William K. Reilly
Administrator, Environmental Protection Agency

Many scientists now understand that loading an animal with a chemical for a lifetime, then counting tumors and feeding a mathematical extrapolation model does not necessarily predict the chemical's potential for causing cancer in humans. In the early days of risk assessment, this modeling approach was the only game in town. It combined some animal data, statistics and mathematical extrapolation to evaluate what chemicals [have] a potential to produce a specific human health effect. This combination process in its many forms became the basis for science policy. *Scientists now understand that the laboratory rodent is not a small human* [emphasis added].

Vernon Houk, M.D.

The implications of this finding go beyond the mere changes in tumor incidence and the impact of this change on EPA's current risk assessment procedures. . . . [They] also indicate that overly conservative assumptions of human cancer risk, such as those inherent in EPA's present potency factor, are not warranted.

Robert Squire, Ph.D., D.M.V.
Dioxin Pathology Working Group
member [one of the original pathologists who had
declared dioxin a major carcinogen after the 1978 study]

If it's a carcinogen, it's a very weak carcinogen and Federal policy needs to reflect that. . . . The effects of EPA's exaggerated risk models is very often to force massive expenditures of money on minuscule risks.

Vernon Houk, M.D.

Dioxin isn't the only chemical regulated on the basis of animal studies; in fact, most are, and that includes the nearly 200 chemicals regulated by the outrageously expensive 1990 Clean Air Act. Interestingly, all are significantly less dangerous than dioxin, as judged by the same animal risk model that has been challenged by the recent findings. If EPA proceeds to regulate dioxin based on human studies—confirming that a mouse is not a little man—they are in effect challenging the basis of the regulation of many other chemicals.

We should encourage EPA to reappraise dioxin expeditiously, pushing forward, then, for other chemicals to be similarly reassessed. The social and economic savings for dioxin-associated industries alone would be momentous: an appropriate downgrading of dioxin's toxicity and a change in relevant public policy, for example, would save the paper and pulp industry an estimated one billion dollars in cleanup costs alone.

It's too late to save the $138 million that the federal government already spent at Times Beach—and it may be too late to save the further costs of the clean-up, estimated at $118 million. The past handling of Times Beach—branding it a toxic waste site—may unfortunately demand present and future remediation.

But we shouldn't waste the $400 million the federal government has spent carefully studying dioxin. In the words of Dr. Houk: "That and other research has given us the science base for good scientific judgments. Now let us have the common sense to use it."

Polychlorinated Biphenyls (PCBs)

Polychlorinated biphenyls (PCBs) had a wide variety of industrial uses in the United States from 1929 to the late 1970s. Their commercial production was then discontinued because of concern about PCB buildup in the environment. This environmental contamination was largely the result of disposal practices now known to have been unwise. PCBs persist for long periods of time in the environment, so we are still dealing with the consequences of past disposal practices.

One place where PCBs tend to accumulate is in fish, particularly those species which eat other fish and accumulate PCBs from their prey in their bodies. On May 22, 1984, the FDA announced that the tolerance level of PCBs in edible fish would be reduced from 5 to 2 parts per million. The commercial fishing industry claimed that they would suffer economic losses with no reasonable expectation that the public health would be improved. The Acting Commissioner of the FDA, on the other hand, claimed that chronic exposure to PCBs in the diet posed a potential risk of liver cancer.

The PCB issue is complex, and it involves many health and environmental considerations other than cancer. Our discussion here will focus only on the potential cancer risk that might be posed by these substances. While this is only one part of the PCB problem, it is the one that caught the public eye, and it was used by FDA to justify its decision about fish.

Do the animal tests on PCBs indicate that they are potent or particularly dangerous carcinogens? No. In fact, it is uncertain whether they cause cancer at all. One study, which was very widely publicized, suggested that PCBs might cause an increase in liver cancer in rats. However, the results of this study have been questioned by many scientists. Another study, on mice, showed only limited and restricted evidence for a carcinogenic effect of a particular PCB compound. Other studies in the mouse and rat have failed to show an increase in liver cancer, and studies in other species have shown no evidence of cancer. Furthermore, an independent researcher who reexamined the slides from the "positive" rat study failed to find any evidence of cancer in the animals' tissues.

What about human evidence? There have been several large studies of workers in the electrical industry who had extensive, longterm exposure to PCBs. Although these individuals had far greater levels of PCBs in their bodies than the general public (even the fish-eating general public) does, no significant adverse health effects were reported except for occasional skin irritations that disappeared quickly. There was no evidence of an increase in liver cancer. Also, during the decades when PCB levels in the U.S. environment were rising, the liver cancer rate in the U.S. was going down.

There have also been studies of people who had higher than usual exposures to PCBs because they ate a lot of fish. A significant correlation between blood PCB levels and the quantity of fish consumed was observed. But an evaluation of the health histories and current health problems of the study subjects did not reveal any differences between the fish eaters and non-fish eaters.

What about substitutes for PCBs? Although we are not evaluating the whole PCB issue here, it's worth mentioning that the alternative materials to PCBs are not without problems. The most important use for PCBs was in electrical equipment, where their flame resistant characteristics were badly needed. Substitute materials do work electrically, but they are often less efficient and many of them present fire hazards. There is concern that the replacement of PCBs with less fire-resistant substitutes may involve the replacement of a hypothetical health risk from PCBs with a product certain to lead to an increased fire hazard.

Did the FDA's tightening of the tolerance level for PCBs

in fish really reduce our risk of liver cancer? There's no reason to think so, since there's no evidence that fish eaters (or even individuals with very high occupational PCB exposures) were at increased risk of liver cancer in the first place. It's more likely that the only result of the FDA action was the condemnation of a lot of nutritious and perfectly edible food, with economic costs to the fishing industry and consumers, and without benefit to public health.

Does Your Cellular Phone or Alarm Clock Give You Cancer?

Cellular phones, alarm clocks, hair dryers, video display terminals (your computer screen), and walkietalkies share at least one thing in common: they emit extremely low frequency levels of electromagnetic energy. In 1993, we've all read—and subsequently are worrying—that this causes cancer.

Electric and magnetic fields are found throughout nature and in all living things. Recall that a compass works because the earth has a magnetic field, created by flowing charges in the earth's molten interior.

There are electric and magnetic fields wherever there is electric power. The electric fields result simply from the strength of the charge. The higher the voltage, the stronger the electric field. It is the motion of the charge that creates magnetic fields. As with electrical fields, the stronger currents produce stronger fields. Any electrical device, such as a hair dryer, that is plugged into a wall socket and turned on generates both electric and magnetic fields. Turned off but left plugged in, that hair dryer will still have an electric field but will no longer have a magnetic field because the charges are not moving. Unlike the electric field, the strength of the magnetic field will change with the setting chosen. When the dryer is operated on high heat setting and draws more current, the magnetic field is greater than when the dryer is on a lower heat setting and drawing less current.

People have become worried about high-voltage transmission lines because they have heard that the magnitude of the electric field is determined by voltage, and that electric fields are most intense nearest high-voltage transmission lines.

The electromagnetic force from any type of electrical power source is actually a type of radiation. That's where the fear comes in. What most people don't understand, however, is that this type of radiation is at the very low end of the electromagnetic spectrum, very distinct from high-energy and high-frequency forms of radiation such as x-rays and cosmic radiation, which carry a significant cancer risk in sufficient doses. Electromagnetic forces are referred to as extremely low frequency radiation, or simply as ELF. They carry too little energy to break chemical bonds or to deposit significant heat in tissue.

The strength of the electric and magnetic fields associated with power lines, wiring, and appliances depends on several factors in addition to the voltage. Trees and houses serve as effective barriers, as does furniture inside the home. In addition, the strength of the field diminishes very quickly with increasing distance.

HEALTH STUDIES FOUND INCONCLUSIVE

At this time it is most accurate to say that no study has ever confirmed that ELF is a cause of human cancer, contrary to what we have all been led to believe. *The Journal of the American Medical Association (JAMA)* wrote in 1992: "It is premature to conclude that ELF poses a risk to humans." Let's look at the evidence.

Brain Cancer. Richard Adamson, Ph.D., director of the National Cancer Institute's (NCI) Division of Cancer Etiology said in 1993: "To date, there have been no definitive studies linking cellular telephones to brain cancer, and there is no need to panic. Studies under way at NCI and others supported by NCI funds will provide information to clarify this concern."

When the cellular phone–brain cancer risk first hit the press, not only did people stop using their cellular phones, but the associated stock prices took a temporary nose dive. And then Quantum Laboratories of Renton, Washington, started marketing a $49.95 product they promised would deflect the phones' radio emissions, "Cellguard." Company officials said they had already developed the device, but came to market with it sooner than expected because "We [didn't] want to miss the emotion of the moment to too much of a degree."

Childhood Leukemia. At least six studies have attempted to find a childhood cancer/electromagnetic forces (EMF) link, comparing children from homes with higher EMF to those of children whose homes had much lower EMF levels. One found no increased risk of cancer; five found a risk ratio from 1.4 for all types of cancer to 3.7 for central nervous system tumors. Experts note that while the most carefully conducted study did find a higher incidence of cancers in higher EMF homes, there may have been some other factor present at the same time as EMF exposure. For example, traffic density was always higher in cases with the EMF/cancer connection. *JAMA,* in 1992, concluded that results are basically conflicting and studies suffer from bias. Also consider that while there has been a tremendous increase in our use of electrical power over the last thirty years, there has not been an increase in the occurrence of childhood leukemias during that same time period. Total per capita electrical power generation, in fact, has increased tenfold since 1940 and per capita residential consumption twentyfold. At the same time, the age-adjusted cancer rate for the whole population has actually been declining (when one removes tobacco-associated cancer deaths).

OCCUPATIONAL EXPOSURE TO EMF

Leukemia. In the United States, at least twelve studies have been undertaken to investigate this claim. All have been positive, with risk ranging from 1.4 to 3.2 for all leukemias considered together. One of these studies, by Matanoski and colleagues at Johns Hopkins University in Baltimore, also revealed a higher incidence for several other cancers, including those of the gastrointestinal system, prostate, and brain. Of eight studies conducted in other countries, two showed no association between leukemia and field exposure. Six did uncover a positive association, with risk ratios varying between 1.3 and 3.8. Overall, though, *JAMA* concluded that studies are conflicting and inconclusive. Job title alone, for example, was taken as the sole evidence of exposure in some studies.

Brain cancer. At least sixteen studies have investigated this association, with five studies focusing on this topic exclusively. These five were all in the occupational setting (with higher than normal levels of exposure, as we discussed in chapter 9); all found some connection, with relative risks ranging widely from 1.5 to 8. Two of the most respected researchers in this field, Nair and Morgan, point out that while the brain tumor-electrical-worker connection seems real, the cause may not be EMFs, but some other factor. Electrical workers are simultaneously exposed to other agents, such as chemicals, which may be the culprit. Indeed, five occupational studies conducted in Sweden failed to find an excess risk for cancer of the brain in electrical workers.

The final—and very telling—point about EMF and cancer is that the EMF we are talking about is many times smaller than the natural amount present in our body's cells. Yale University physicist Robert Adair, Ph.D., an outspoken critic of EMF research says:

> Anyone who would believe that EMFs could promote cancer would believe in perpetual motion or cold fusion. In my mind, this falls into the realm of aberrant science— very difficult experience, very marginal data that are never quite reproducible, and results that don't increase proportionally when the factor increases.

Do Pesticides Cause Breast Cancer?

Breast cancer is undeniably a major health problem in the United States. Not only is it the most frequently diagnosed form of cancer, but breast cancer is the second leading cause of cancer death among American women. (In 1987, lung cancer surpassed breast cancer as the major cause of cancer death among women in the United States.) According to American Cancer Society estimates, in 1992, 180,000 women were diagnosed with breast cancer and 46,000 women died as a result of the disease.

Although most scientists agree that breast cancer is an essential area of future research, many feel that an undue portion of funding will be directed toward the search for hypothetical environmental causes of the disease. These scientists' fears are apparently well justified. The 1993 NIH reauthorization bill, passed by the House of Representatives this past March, requires the National Cancer Institute to conduct a study of environmental risk factors in Long Island, New York. (This area has received considerable media attention recently because the rates of breast cancer in this area are higher than the national average for the disease.) Representative Henry Waxman (D-California) added to this authorization bill an amendment directing NCI and the National Institute of Environmental Health Sciences to "launch a case-control study to assess biological markers for environmental and other risk factors contributing to the incidence of breast cancer in the counties of Nassau and Suffolk in the state of New York."

CONTRARY FINDINGS BY THE CDC

The allocation of funds toward the search for environmental causes seems particularly surprising because of recent findings of the Centers for Disease Control and Prevention. In February 1992, the CDC agreed to provide "technical assistance" to the New York State Department of Health (NYSDOH) in the investigation of the high incidence of breast cancer among women of Long Island, New York. The objectives of the study, according to the panel members, were as follows:

> We reviewed the concerns of the community, the literature on breast cancer and environmental factors, incidence and mortality data, and studies related to breast cancer on Long Island. Using data collected in previous studies from women on Long Island, we performed an analysis to compare the incidence rate for Nassau county with that of the neighboring Suffolk county, taking into account the prevalence of known risk factors for breast cancer in the two counties.

The analysis conducted by this panel of experts revealed that the high incidence of breast cancer within Nassau county can be explained by the demographics of the women living in this area. The women of Nassau county have a higher prevalence of certain known risk factors including a history of benign breast disease, certain reproductive history traits and ethnic origin. When the researchers controlled for these variables, the women did not appear to have an extraordinarily high rate for the disease.

Despite the findings of the CDC panel, the misguided search for unseen environmental links to the disease continues. A recent study in the Journal of the National Cancer Institute (JNCI) is eliciting considerable attention. Alarmists are stating that this study may provide some of the first evidence for an association between breast cancer and certain environmental causes.

DDT-BREAST CANCER CONNECTION

The study, titled "Blood Levels of Organochlorine Residues and Risk of Breast Cancer," was designed to determine whether the pesticide DDT and PCBs are associated with increased breast cancer risk in women. The principal investigators were Dr. Mary S. Wolff and her colleagues at the Mount Sinai Medical School. Fifty-eight cases and 171 matched control subjects were selected from a population of New York City women. According to researchers, their data showed a "fourfold increase in the relative risk of breast cancer for an elevation of serum DDE." (DDE is the by-product of DDT found in the body.) No similar association could be made for PCBs.

The findings of this study, though worth pursuing, should be looked at only as the results of a preliminary investigation. However, the media and environmental groups have already begun to use this study as evidence of the link between organochlorine, pesticides and cancer. A series of articles appeared in major newspapers across the country with such titles as "First DDT Link to Breast Cancer Reported."

Also troubling was the manner in which the article was presented in JNCI. An accompanying editorial, written by David J. Hunter and Karl T. Kelsey, over-emphasized the importance of the study. Although the authors of this editorial initially acknowledge some of the flaws of the Wolff study, such as small sample size, they later state that the findings have far-reaching implications:

> Because the findings of Wolff et al. may have extraordinary global implications for the prevention of breast cancer, their study should serve as a wake-up call for further urgent research.

Since 1990, approximately 12,045 papers on various aspects of breast cancer have been indexed by the National Library of Medicine. Is it fair or reasonable to hold the Wolff study so far above the numerous other research articles on breast cancer? The authors of the JNCI editorial apparently belittle the contributions made by many other respected scientists and cancer researchers. The suggestive language used in the editorial leads the reader to believe that the Wolff study is the only valid research available on the safety and carcinogenicity of DDT. In fact, a vast body of research already exists on DDT and its effects on human health.

The Facts about DDT. The initial concern about DDT stemmed from the theory that the pesticide induced tumors and reproductive problems in some animal species. It was believed that the chemical caused eggshell thinning in certain types of birds. Reports followed that DDT was a cancer promoter in mice, and that the chemical accumulated in the food chain with storage in the body fat of mammals. All of these concerns lead to a popular outcry to ban DDT. In 1972, the chemical was officially banned in the United States.

However, reports followed that DDT was not the public hazard described by the media. In 1984, the World Health Organization (WHO) and the Food and Agriculture Organization of the United Nations (FAO) issued a report which elucidated many of the facts about DDT.

The FAO and WHO report concluded that DDT was in fact, *not a carcinogen in mice.* Although the chemical was found to induce liver nodules, these tumors did not invade adjacent tissues or metastasize. The liver tumors could also not be induced in other rodent species.

The same FAO and WHO report concluded that DDT was also not a carcinogen in man or any other species, such as hamster, rat or monkey. The results of the report were based on a review of the vast body of literature on the cancer causing potential of the chemical.

Scientists feared the DDT—egg thinning connection because such an effect in animals might indicate that the chemical could also affect the human reproductive cycle. Recent research implicates fluctuations in hormonal levels, particularly estrogen, as being associated with increased breast cancer risk. Any chemical labeled "estrogenic" is deemed worthy of further investigation by cancer researchers. Eggshell thinning and reproductive failure in birds is seen by some investigators as a marker of DDT's "estrogenic effects." However, in most studies, eggshell thinning has not been associated with estrogenicity. The evidence of DDT's effects on human reproductive hormones is shaky at best.

Real Implications of the DDT—Breast Cancer Association. The results of the Wolff study warrant some further investigation. A larger study is needed to substantiate its findings. In fact, the Wolff study raises more questions than it answers. Some questions definitely require further consideration:

- Association is not the same as causation. Thousands of biochemical changes result in the body due to the development of cancer. Is the elevated level of DDT a result or the cause of breast cancer in these cases?

- DDT was banned in the United States twenty years ago. Where is the practical potential for cancer prevention in the United States in further investigating the health hazards of the chemical?

- DDT use worldwide is greater today than in 1972. Is one of the "global implications" of Wolff's paper that DDT should be banned worldwide? (Discontinuing the use of DDT could lead to a dramatic increase in insect-borne disease.)

- Why investigate DDT exposure in New York? DDT was "overused" primarily in the Southern portion of the United States. Is the increased incidence of breast cancer in Long Island related to some "unseen" over-exposure to the chemical? When was this cohort of women exposed? Did the exposure occur in New York? (No data is provided in the Wolff article to suggest when and where the exposure to DDT occurred.)

Redirecting funds from such valuable pursuits as searches for effective treatments, many experts contend, would be a grave mistake. Policy makers need to decide if searching for "toxic phantoms" will be a fruitful endeavor or yet another unnecessary burden on our public health research budget. The "wake-up call" should be to those who can prevent a disproportionate amount of research dollars from going into relatively low priority fields at the expense of programs that directly benefit the breast cancer patient.

How Many People Died of Cancer at Love Canal, New York?

Love Canal is an icon of the environmental movement. It is the story of half truths and political motivations.

But it was never a cause of human cancer.

Former Governor Hugh Carey summarizes the situation by saying: "Love Canal is the story of people trying to create an issue where there wasn't one."

Love Canal, New York, became a national media event in the 1970s when thirty-year-old chemical wastes buried there began to leak several years after irresponsible excavation.

But despite the chemical leakage, there haven't been any cases of human cancer (or of birth defects). The lack of evidence for damage to human health was confirmed by a thorough analysis of all published and unpublished studies by the Committee on Environmental Epidemiology of the National Research Council, who published their review in 1991.

Without a doubt, no one wants another Love Canal; we must strive to manage the benefits of technology safely and appropriately. We must also acknowledge that the heavily industrialized areas of this country are no longer pristine. That doesn't mean we should simply write them off, or declare them a cause of human cancer because we are repulsed by them, as the environmentalists have tried to fervently to do with Love Canal.

Are Nuclear Power Plants
Increasing Our Cancer Burden?

As more and more intricate technologies have found their way to the market during the twentieth century, Americans have become increasingly concerned with the concept of health risks. Many now believe that modern man has created a world that is inherently more risky than ever before. Radiation associated with nuclear power operations, for example, is widely viewed as one of the greatest risks to human life and the environment.

Why are nuclear power and radiation of such great concern to so many Americans? There is no simple answer. An enormous amount of information about nuclear technology is available to the public, but deciding on whom or what to believe may be quite confusing when one is confronted with conflicting accounts of the same issue.

If nuclear power plant operations substantially increased overall radiation exposure to people, the possible adverse effects of the radiation would be an important health concern. But the average dose to a U.S. resident from the one hundred ten reactors currently in commercial operation is estimated at less than one millirem per year, substantially less than the 20,000 millirads which studies have found to be hazardous. People living close to a nuclear plant are exposed to a radiation dose ranging from a few millirads in the plant's immediate vicinity to 0.05 millirads at locations fifty miles from a plant. Nuclear energy produces little real impact on human health or the environment compared to the burning of fossil fuels. The health risk imposed on those living near a fossil fuel plant is significant and well documented, as opposed to the imagined risks of living in the vicinity of a nuclear power plant.

Indeed, epidemiological studies of people living in these areas confirms that there is no health risk associated with living near a nuclear plant. Cancer incidence and mortality studies in the vicinity of nuclear installations in England and Wales during the period 1959–1980 concluded that there has been no general increase in cancer mortality. The only exceptions were leukemia in young people and a small increase in multiple myeloma and Hodgkin's disease in people twenty-five to seventy-four years of age. A companion study compared mortality due to leukemia and Hodgkin's disease in people who lived near potential sites to that of people who lived near existing sites and found no difference in mortality between the two groups. They hypothesized that existing and potential sites might share unrecognized risk factors other than the radiation.

The National Cancer Institute (NCI) also investigated cancer mortality among populations living near nuclear facilities, with a special focus on childhood leukemias in light of the British findings. Their study, released September 19, 1990, showed no general increased risk of death from cancer for people living in 107 U.S. counties or closely adjacent to sixty-two nuclear facilities, including fifty-two commercial nuclear power plants, nine Department of Energy research and weapons plants, and one commercial fuel-reprocessing plant. Deaths from sixteen types of cancer, including leukemia, were compared to cancer rates in 292 similar counties without nuclear facilities. According to John Boice, Sc.D., chief of NCI's Radiation Epidemiology Branch,

From the data at hand, there was no convincing evidence of any increased risk of death from any of the cancers we surveyed due to living near nuclear facilities.

Nuclear industry workers receive an average exposure of 400 millirems per year which, over a forty-seven-year working life, may reduce their life expectancy by ten days. By comparison, occupational accidents reduce life expectancy for the *average* U.S. worker by seventy-four days, and for miners and construction workers by 300 days. Occupational diseases, stress, and other factors reduce life expectancy in many occupations by 800 to 1,400 days. Spending one's entire life as a radiation worker increases one's risk of dying of cancer by about 4.94 percent.

Experts, however, caution that this 4.94 percent excess may be falsely elevated. Says Geoffrey R. Howe, Ph.D., of the National Cancer Institute of Canada:

This interpretation requires considerable caution. The observed excess incidence of cancer is limited to a relatively short period of time at the end of the follow-up interval, to an excess incidence of leukemia primarily in one dose group, and to an excess incidence of lung cancer, which is difficult to interpret in the absence of smoking data.

Dr. Howe concludes with:

It is somewhat ironic that public concern over the potential hazards of normally operating nuclear facilities receives much greater attention than the far greater risks imposed by such voluntary lifestyle factors as smoking, drinking and diet.

People living near the highly publicized Three Mile Island nuclear power plant accident received an average dose of one millirad. This amounts to one chance in seven million of getting a fatal cancer from that exposure; or, putting it another way, their increased risk of death is the same as they would face in four extra street crossings or four puffs on a cigarette. In fact, the risks of evacuation from the Harrisburg area were greater than the risk from radiation exposure for the residents who remained.

WHAT HAPPENED AT THREE MILE ISLAND?

During the early morning hours of March 29, 1979, a pump responsible for transporting water to the steam generator malfunctioned in the Three Mile Island (TMI) nuclear facility in eastern Pennsylvania. This incident was the first in a series of human and mechanical errors which make up what is widely considered to be the worst U.S. nuclear power accident in history. Antinuclear groups point to the TMI experience as the ultimate proof of the danger of nuclear power, but a close look at what actually happened reveals that the safety apparatus built into a nuclear power plant does in fact ensure that the public health and environment will be protected in the event of a mishap.

TMI is in fact a disaster—an economic one, causing more than one billion dollars' worth of damage. Fortunately, it was not the health disaster the public thought it was. Although the consequences of such economic disasters are enormous and not to be ignored, the most important consequences of this or any other accident are the effects on human health. How close did we come to a catastrophic release of high amounts of radioactive materials?

Some have said that if a reactor core is heated uncontrollably and reaches approximately five thousand degrees Fahrenheit, it might melt through the bottom of the containment vessel, resulting in an enormous, health-threatening release of radiation. Before TMI, some believed that if the core of a reactor was uncovered for even a short period of time (more than a few minutes), a "meltdown" could not be avoided. At TMI the core was uncovered, except for steam, for a number of hours, yet a meltdown did not occur. The emergency water-cooling system was mistakenly turned off, yet the steam in the vessel served as a sufficient coolant to keep the core from melting.

The official body established by President Carter to study TMI, the Kemeny Commission, concluded that damage was contained despite many human errors and a few mechanical failures. Its report concluded:

- If a meltdown would have occurred (and it wasn't even imminent), radiological releases would not have been increased significantly.

- The airtight building did not fail. More importantly, it would have not failed if there had been a meltdown.

- Neither the reactor vessel nor the containment building would have been ruptured by a steam or hydrogen explosion.

- If the complete core had melted down, it probably would not have melted through the concrete base mat of the containment building.

The Kemeny Commission also reassured us that there is absolutely no evidence suggesting that human or animal life was threatened by the accident. Neighbors of the plant received a maximum exposure to 70 millirads and *an average of only 1 millirad due to the TMI malfunction.* To put this into perspective, a person receiving the maximum might have been exposed to more radiation from two medical chest x-rays.

At TMI, despite everything that went wrong, we learned that the backup systems and safeguards built into U.S. designs really work. Before TMI it was generally thought that if temperatures within a reactor core got high enough to melt the fuel, the fuel would melt through the bottom of the containment vessel and result in an enormous, catastrophic release of radiation. At TMI, when the emergency water-cooling system was mistakenly turned off, the core was uncovered and a portion of the fuel did actually melt. But the other safeguards built into the plant kept even this serious accident from threatening the health and safety of the public. The water in the TMI containment building retained virtually 100 percent of the radioactivity, and the building maintained its integrity.

More than a decade after TMI, we understand more clearly than ever that the safety features in nuclear plants are both essential and effective. But, just as important, we are also beginning to understand just how badly America needs nuclear power. It is non-polluting. It doesn't depend on the political stability of other nations thousands of miles away. And, as TMI showed us, it is safe.

AND WHAT HAPPENED AT CHERNOBYL?

On April 26, 1986, a serious accident occurred at the Chernobyl Atomic Power Station in the Soviet Union. Serious damage to the core and a fire were followed by the release of a large amount of radioactivity into the environment. Many people were hospitalized for radiation exposure and there were 31 deaths among the firefighters and emergency personnel working directly at the scene. In the aftermath, over 100,000 people had to be evacuated from the area.

Several important factors assure us that this type of accident could not occur in the United States. First of all, the Chernobyl reactor design is unique to power plants used inside the Soviet Union. This design is not at all comparable to commercial reactors in the United States and in other Western countries. Most significantly, the Chernobyl reactor's design makes it unstable during low-power operation; at the time of the accident, the reactor was indeed being operated at low power. Second, multiple operator errors significantly contributed to the escalation of the accident. Operators were performing experiments at the time and made a series of crucial mistakes which resulted in an uncontrollable reaction that destroyed the reactor core and released large amounts of radioactivity. Reassuringly, key Soviet scientists acknowledge the superiority of U.S. designs. Top U.S. nuclear power experts are certain that this type of accident could not happen in a U.S.-style power plant.

Does Air Pollution Contribute to Lung Cancer?

We know that traces of suspected carcinogens, for example benzo(a)pyrene and other polycyclic aromatic hydrocarbons, can be found in our air. Workers in some industries have been exposed to dangerously high concentrations of carcinogens, but at levels many times higher than the levels in ambient air. We are painfully aware that inhalation of asbestos and various ores in industrial situations increases the odds of those workers developing lung cancer. For example, in Germany during the late nineteenth century, environmentally induced lung cancer occurred among uranium miners. Workers in coal mines have been afflicted with a number of respiratory ailments, including lung cancer, as a result of exposure to coal tar and volatile substances released from coal tar such as benzo(a)pyrene. Nickel refiners exposed to chromates and chrome ore dust, and iron ore miners exposed to iron oxide also have an increased risk of developing cancer of the lungs. Thus it is theoretically possible that the cancer-causing agents we breathe each day increase our risk of cancer of the site with which the air is most likely to come in close contact: our lungs.

Unlike cigarette smoking, industrial, and occupational exposure, the potential cancer risk from air pollution concerns all of us. Interest in a possible relationship between community air pollution and cancer has come about for two main reasons: First, certain epidemiological studies suggest that smoking habits cannot fully explain the excess cancer mortality in urban residents. Second, as mentioned above, known carcinogenic agents have been identified in urban air.

Lung cancer *does* occur more often in cities than in rural portions of the country. But, in addition to the air being different in these two types of localities, the people and other community characteristics are different. Of minor, though not insignificant, importance is that cities have more facilities for diagnosing lung cancer. Of somewhat more significance is that more city dwellers may in the past have had some type of occupational exposure which predisposed them to developing lung cancer.

One EPA investigation revealed, in fact, that residents in highly industrial areas are at no greater health risk from air pollutants than are people in rural areas. For two days 350 residents of Elizabeth and Bayonne, New Jersey, wore monitors sensitive enough to register the effect of a visit to the dry cleaner. These monitors revealed that the dosage of volatile air toxics from industrial plants was but a fraction of the total inhaled, anywhere from one-half to one-seventieth, depending on the pollutant. The total intake of industrial pollutants was no greater for the urban dwellers than for those in a comparison farm town in North Dakota.

Of specific concern has been the possibility that airborne asbestos, a known human carcinogen, could be posing a general cancer hazard. As discussed in chapter 8, asbestos can be inhaled by persons who install or repair dry walls, roofing, flooring, automobile brakes and clutches, or home heating and plumbing systems, placing them at risk of developing lung disease. But exposure to asbestos in the outdoor environment probably doesn't contribute to lung cancer, as summarized by Drs. Carl M. Shy and Robert J. Struba in *Cancer Epidemiology and Prevention*, it is likely that "low ambient asbestos levels and levels encountered during incidental nonoccupational exposure to asbestos products constitute a very low risk of lung cancer to the general population." Furthermore, the Advisory Committee on Asbestos

Cancers to the director of the International Agency for Research on Cancer concluded, after studying the effects of low-level occupational exposure to asbestos, "Excess lung cancer is not detectable when occupational exposures to asbestos have been low, and these exposures have almost certainly been greater than those of the public from general air pollution."

So, then, does air pollution cause cancer? The conclusions of most scientists, offered from the early 1980s through the early 1990s, are that air pollution probably contributes very little to the cancer burden:

> The assertion that ambient air pollution is a risk factor for cancer, particularly lung cancer is . . . unwarranted.
>
> Carl M. Shy and Robert J. Stuba

> . . . air pollution was not found to be a great culprit in causing lung cancer.
>
> American Cancer Society

John D. Graham, associate professor of Policy and Decision Sciences at Harvard School of Public Health, told Congress in September 1989 that if air pollution contributes to lung cancer, that contribution is most incidental:

> While there is a logical basis for public health concern, there is no direct evidence that outdoor exposures to toxic air pollutants are responsible for a significant fraction of disease or mortality. The levels of toxics that people breathe in daily life are typically several factors of ten smaller than the levels that have been studied by scientists. Based

on a study of 65 toxic air pollutants, the EPA estimates that up to 3,000 additional cancers from [air toxics] may occur each year in the United States. By way of comparison, keep in mind that 900,000 new cases of cancer are detected in the United States each year.

But Graham goes on to qualify these estimates:

The EPA's widely quoted cancer risk estimates should be treated with caution because they are based on some questionable assumptions—for example, that humans are as sensitive as the most sensitive tested animal species, and that any human exposure to a carcinogen, no matter how small, results in some increase in cancer risk. While these are prudent assumptions to make in the absence of sound data, the EPA has not always been responsive about revising its assumptions in light of scientific advances. For example, the EPA's risk assessment for benzene, for-maldehyde, gasoline vapor, and perchloroethylene are scientifically outdated and need to be revised.

Does Polluted Water Cause Cancer?

Theoretically, it is possible that a water supply could contain enough cancer-causing agents to increase cancer risk in a population exposed to it for a lifetime. For example, our ex-perience with the radium dial workers indicates that human beings ingesting large quantities of radioactive material (in this case, swallowing the paint used to create luminescent watch dials) had a significantly higher rate of bone cancer. Thus, for example, if our water supply was contaminated with sufficiently higher quantities of radium, it seems likely that this would elevate cancer mortality. The questions, then, are, Are there carcinogens in our water supply? If so, are they there at high enough levels to cause cancer?

Given the fact that we now have analytical techniques that permit us to detect chemicals at concentrations well below one part per billion (that is the equivalent of one square foot in thirty-six square miles, one bad apple in two million barrels, or one pinch of salt in ten tons of potato chips), the answer to the question whether we can detect carcinogens in our water supply is yes. The carcinogens we speak of here are those which cause cancer in laboratory experiments—and, in at least one case, a substance which has been shown to cause cancer when inhaled by humans, namely, asbestos. The more important question for practical effect is, At what level do these carcinogens occur and what is the evidence linking them to cancer?

The level of carcinogens in the American water supply is extremely low and, according to most public health experts, poses no significant risk of cancer to the human population. Doll and Peto, in their classic work *The Causes of Cancer*, looked at the question of water pollution and cancer and concluded, "It is not plausible that any material percentage of the total number of cancers in the whole United States derives from this source."

One concern that they did have was the presence of asbestos in some local water supplies; for example, those of New Orleans. Asbestos, as reviewed in chapter 8, has been clearly shown to increase risk of lung cancer, mesothelioma, and other diseases when inhaled, and there is the suggestion that some asbestos workers were at greater risk of gastrointestinal cancer because of ingestion of dust through the respiratory passages. Furthermore, asbestos fibers are present in varying concentrations in surface waters (and subsequently drinking waters) around the country. They enter water supplies mainly from construction products such as cement and from mining activities, as noted in the previously mentioned case of Duluth, Minnesota.

Schottenfeld and Fraumeni, in what is considered the essential textbook on cancer epidemiology, *Cancer Epidemiology and Prevention,* reviewed the literature available on asbestos exposure from water, and concluded that "most epidemiologic studies of populations served by water containing high concentrations of asbestos have failed to yield . . . conclusive results [of an association between asbestos in water and cancer.]" Stating that some evidence suggests a positive correlation between asbestos and cancer, the authors recommend continued research in this area.

There is some evidence that drinking water with high levels of the metal arsenic may cause skin cancer. It is based mainly on studies conducted in Taiwan, where waters contain arsenic in much higher concentrations than do those in the United States. Schottenfeld and Fraumeni state, "On the basis of existing evidence, it is not possible to conclude that arsenic, or any other metal present in drinking water, causes cancer in humans by ingestion of ambient trace amounts. However, the broad distribution of these metals in drinking water indicates a need for further study in this area."

Experts at the National Cancer Institute, led by Herman Kraybill, Ph.D., are compulsively studying the water-cancer connection. This committee says there are too many uncontrolled variants to draw any conclusions. They concluded that:

While the experimental and epidemiologic studies provide some presumptive evidence, one cannot establish, with any degree of assurance as yet, any causality relevant to cancer from these micropollutants. There is serious concern, however, about those contaminants with the realization that [they] may contribute to the total cancer burden. Thus, control and reduction technologies in water treatment are recommended.

The water-cancer question challenges science for two main reasons: First, it is difficult to detect and measure trace contaminants. Second, science doesn't understand how such contaminants work together, or cancel each other, in the process of causing cancer. Future study can and will supply answers to many of the unknowns that cloud the picture today. But the evidence collected to date clearly refutes the claim that we as a society are subject to a dangerous risk of cancer from drinking water.

SHOULD YOU STOP DRINKING CHLORINATED WATER?

Chlorinated drinking water offers tremendous health benefits. Since chlorination was introduced in 1908 as a disinfectant for drinking water, the incidence of water-borne infectious diseases—typhoid, cholera, polio, and hepatitis, for example—has dropped dramatically.

Concern about chlorination arose in the 1970s when scientists discovered that byproducts formed in the process of disinfecting water with chlorine caused cancer in laboratory animals. More recent population-based studies consistently found an increased risk of bladder and rectal cancer in humans who drink chlorinated water, noting a 21 percent increase in bladder cancer and a 38 percent increase in rectal cancer. (Researchers found no increased risk of brain, breast, colon, rectal, esophageal, kidney, liver, lung, or pancreatic cancer.) Before you eschew your public water supply, it is critically important to put these risks into perspective.

First, let's look at how these increases translate into numbers of people affected. According to the American Cancer Society (ACS), there are approximately 45,000 new cases of rectal cancer each year. Just 18 percent, or 8,100 cases are associated with drinking chlorinated water. The ACS estimates that there are 51,000 new cases of bladder cancer each year, with nine percent or 4,644 attributable to chlorinated water. In contrast, say experts at the National Cancer Institute (NCI), the more significant causes of bladder cancer are cigarette smoking and occupational exposure, responsible for 70 percent of such cancers in men and 40 percent in women.

The most critical perspective, however, lies in considering the consequences of not chlorinating water. The World Health Organization estimates that 25,000 people die each day from diseases carried by inadequately sanitized water. In a year, that's 9.1 million deaths. The risk of death from not chlorinating water, then, is of gargantuan proportions when compared with the chances of contracting cancer from drinking chlorinated water. One must also bear in mind that although contracting cancer may be devastating, many cancers—including rectal and bladder cancers—are treatable or even curable.

Finally, advises the NCI, it is still not clear which compounds in chlorinated water are responsible for the cancer association. In fact, it may not be the chlorine or chlorination byproducts causing the excess cancers. As with any population-based study, finding an association between some factor—such as chlorinated water and increased disease, in this case rectal and bladder cancers—does not necessarily mean that the factor is responsible. Chlorination may only serve as a marker for some other aspect of drinking water quality or an associated geographic or demographic variable that causes the cancers.

I hope it's clear that you *shouldn't* stop drinking chlorinated water to prevent cancer. The benefit simply isn't worth the risk.

Why You Shouldn't Worry Too Much About Animal Tests

Those who translate scientific findings into news reports, and, worse yet, into regulatory actions often seem to be operating under the assumption that if a substance causes cancer under any circumstances in any animal, it must cause cancer under normal circumstances in human use. Yet, as discussed in chapter 1, there is absolutely no basis for this conclusion. In fact, we know that it is false. Scientists and regulators, recognizing the need for prudence and acknowledging the limitations of scientific knowledge, have deliberately stacked the deck against substances under investigation. They have treated these substances as guilty until proven innocent and made it virtually impossible for anything to be proven innocent.

It is crucial to remember that in evaluating the animal test results used to determine whether a substance is a carcinogen, scientists and regulators have deliberately:

- chosen the most sensitive species, strain, and sex of animal

- used the highest possible dose of the test chemical, even though this may cause abnormal changes in the animal's metabolic processes

- assumed that the response (cancer production) to a chemical is directly proportional to dose, when in fact careful tests on a number of chemicals have shown that this is rarely true, and that low doses of a chemical are often much less hazardous than this assumption would predict

- given greater credence to positive animal studies than to negative animal or human evidence

- assumed that the question "Does it cause cancer?" has a simple yes/no answer, and ignored evidence about the potency of a carcinogen that might provide perspective on the degree of risk that a particular substance might pose.

These assumptions were made in good faith and with the best intentions—to protect human health. But they were based on a fundamental and usually unmentioned basic premise: that substances that produce positive results in animal cancer tests are few in number and generally man-made in origin. With this understanding, a prudent and sensible response to the discovery that a substance to which people were exposed showed carcinogenic activity in animal tests would be to eliminate all human exposure to it. Indeed, it was hoped at one time that a substantial reduction in cancer could be achieved by the simple means of banning a comparatively small number of man-made chemicals. Certainly, some substances might have been unnecessarily banned, with resulting losses to the economy and the consumer, but such decisions could be expected to be few in number and clearly outweighed by the benefit of eliminating our exposure to carcinogens.

Scientists have learned, however, that substances producing positive results in animal cancer tests are actually numerous rather than few, and that a very substantial number of naturally occurring substances produce positive responses in these tests. As we learned, many of these natural carcinogens are normally present in our food. Human exposure to such natural carcinogens cannot in general be readily eliminated; a normal diet invariably contains them. They are often present in amounts much greater than the amounts of man-made carcinogens to which we are exposed. In some instances, they are as potent or more potent than man-made carcinogens. Yet we seem to coexist with them rather well. Indeed, while we have been able to identify a substantial number of natural carcinogens in our diet, we don't have much evidence as yet that any of these matters very much in affecting human cancer rates.

Putting Carcinogens into Perspective

In order to put the accumulating information about natural and man-made carcinogens into proper perspective, we must accept one basic principle: a carcinogen should be evaluated and regulated on the basis of its hazard to humans, not its natural or man-made origin. Some people have challenged this principle on several grounds. Let's examine their arguments carefully.

First, it has been argued that man-made chemicals are

particularly dangerous because they are new, and humans have not had a chance to adapt to them during evolution. This position seems to have little merit. If the argument were valid, then laboratory animals, which have also evolved in the presence of nature's carcinogens, shouldn't get cancer when exposed to them. But they do get cancer—that's how these substances were identified as carcinogens in the first place.

Second, it has been argued that man-made carcinogens are particularly dangerous because they might interact with each other in deleterious ways. This type of interaction is certainly possible. But the same possibility holds for natural carcinogens, and interactions involving natural substances are actually more likely, since their number, variety, and amount are greater.

Third, it has been argued that we should continue to focus our cancer prevention efforts on man-made carcinogens, since we can fairly easily stop using them, while there is little or nothing that we can do about natural carcinogens. This attitude is defeatist and counterproductive. We should be focusing our attentions on the most important hazards, not the easiest ones to correct. Should we ignore a natural carcinogen if there is evidence that it is a real threat to our health, just because it is difficult to regulate it? Of course not. And in fact, we do not ignore such substances. Aflatoxins, for instance, are natural and they are a real threat if we permit them to contaminate our foods in substantial amounts. In the United States, we make great efforts to prevent such contamination and these efforts are successful.

It is also important to consider that man-made chemicals are present in our foods and other parts of our environment because they serve some practical purpose, while natural carcinogens are just there. Unless existing alternatives to the man-made chemicals can perform the same function and are not known to be carcinogens, we risk losing the beneficial function altogether.

In order to put the hazards of any carcinogen—natural or manmade—into perspective, we need to evaluate the degree of risk it poses to humans. To do this, we should be asking questions such as the following:

- How potent a carcinogen is it?

- Does it show signs of being a particularly dangerous carcinogen, e.g., causing tumors in many animal species, causing highly lethal tumors, causing tumors that do not occur spontaneously in that type of animal, or producing tumors with a very short lag time?

- Do we know anything about how the response to this substance varies with dose?

- How do the levels of human exposure compare with the levels that have caused cancer in animals?

- Do we have any human evidence on the carcinogenicity of this substance? In particular, do we have evidence on its effects on groups of people exposed to unusually large amounts of it?

- If we eliminate the use of this substance, what benefits do we lose? Are there adequate substitutes? Are the substitutes safer than the chemical under consideration? If there is no safe substitute, do the overall risks of banning the substance exceed the risks of keeping it?

12

Screening for Early Detection of Cancer

According to I. Bernard Weinstein, M.D., of Columbia University Comprehensive Cancer Center, 50 to 80 percent of cancers are preventable by practicing certain habits: not smoking, eating the healthy diet we outlined, avoiding multiple sexual partners, and avoiding infections like hepatitis B and AIDS.

John Higginson, M.D., of the Institute for Healthy Policy Analysis Georgetown University Medical Center in Washington says, on the other hand, that the eliminatory approach—eliminating minute quantities of pollutants in the ambient environment—will have little impact on the cancer burden.

To control cancer, we need to continue studies that help define the causes of cancer; they are indeed the bridges to cancer control. In the best of all worlds, we would like to determine the acceptable exposure levels to potential human carcinogens. But this remains a formidable task, one for which no scientific framework yet exists.

Let's look at the issue of screening, which is essential to detecting cancer early.

The Importance of Early Detection

Most treatments for cancer work much better when used on small cancers or cancers that are not advanced. Doctors measure how far advanced a tumor is by assigning it a "stage," usually I to IV. The stage given depends upon the size of the tumor, whether it has spread to nearby lymph nodes, and whether it has spread to distant sites such as bone or liver. Staging systems vary by specific cancer but generally a Stage I cancer is small and has not spread to regional lymph nodes or distant sites. Stage IV cancers have generally metastasized (spread) to other sites throughout the body. As one can imagine, it is much easier to treat a Stage I disease than a Stage IV disease. For a Stage I cancer it may be possible to surgically remove or locally irradiate every cancer cell and thus effect a cure. If this is not possible, chemotherapy or radiation therapy may be able to eradicate the relatively few remaining cells. For a very few cancers, chemotherapy or radiation alone can cure the disease.

In many cancers, how well a patient does depends greatly upon the stage at which the cancer is detected. Thus, if the disease can be detected at an early stage, there is a much greater chance for cure. This is the purpose of cancer screening: to detect cancers early in their development to provide the patient with a greater chance of cure.

How a Screening Test Is Evaluated

Not all methods for detecting cancer are useful for screening. Several attributes of a test must be evaluated to decide if it should be recommended for screening purposes. First, the test should be able to detect the disease in most people who have it. This is referred to as the sensitivity of the test. In other words, there would be few "false-negatives," i.e., people who were screened negative but actually did have cancer. The fewer cancers a screening test will miss (the fewer false-negatives), the more valuable it will be. No test can be perfect and identify everybody with cancer, but the test should detect at least 30 to 90 percent of the people with the disease.

Another important feature of a screening test is the specificity of the test. This ensures that when the test is positive the person really has the disease. Most tests will have a certain percentage of "false-positives," people who tested positive but who do not actually have the disease. What percentage of false-positives is permissible depends on what is at stake. If, for example, a pathologist who examined biopsy specimens issued many false-positive reports, many patients would be subjected to unnecessary treatment. Fortunately, tissue diagnosis is very accurate, with fewer than 1 percent false-positives. On the other hand, the test for checking stool for trace amounts of blood has a very high false-positive rate. This is acceptable because several other tests are then used to determine the presence of cancer. Few tests are both very specific and very sensitive at the same time, (i.e., low false-negative and false-positive rates). Often one must trade off one for the other.

It is also important to assess the potential risk of any

screening test. Although the overall risks are small, there is obviously much more risk in a colonoscopy (passing a small flexible tube through the colon) than in simply checking the stool for traces of blood. Some risks, such as that from an x-ray or mammogram, are difficult to quantify because, although they exist, they are very small per each test. More subtle risks need to be recognized as well. These include the potential psychological damage caused by identifying a person as possibly having cancer who does not. If the individual had not been screened, the trauma would not have occurred and no benefit resulted from the screening.

Finally, one must consider the financial cost of screening. It is, of course, impossible to put a dollar figure on a human life, but unfortunately we as individuals and as a nation have limited resources. Thus a screening test must be affordable. If all resources were spent on screening for cancer, there would not be enough left to treat the disease itself.

The ideal screening test then would be specific (pick up all those with the disease), sensitive (have few false-positives), low in risk to the person being screened, easy to do and inexpensive. Unfortunately, no test is perfect and each potential screening test must be evaluated by the above criteria to assess its value.

When to Screen for Cancer

Several criteria must be met for a screening test to be useful. First, there must be a reasonable chance of detecting the cancer. If a cancer occurs only in one in a million people, it is unlikely that screening a million people would be feasible to detect just one cancer. Second, the benefit of the screening test or tests must be greater than the potential harm of the screening procedure. It would not make sense to detect a hundred cases of cancer while causing a hundred serious complications from the screening test itself. The cost of the test must also be reasonable. A test which costs an inordinate amount of money would not be feasible for mass screening.

Finally, early detection of the cancer by the screening test must improve the chances of survival. If there is no treatment for a disease or if survival from cancer is no different whether it is detected through screening or when it causes symptoms, there is no benefit from the screening. In other words, if detecting the cancer early is not going to help the patient, there is no reason to screen for the cancer in the first place. This may seem a trivial point, but as discussed below, it has affected the recommendations for lung cancer screening significantly. Determining whether screening affects survival is not simple. Large studies with lengthy follow-up are needed and the costs of such studies can be prohibitive. There is also concern that the apparent benefits of screening may result simply from the fact that it detects cancers earlier than they would normally be found. Patients would then appear to do better not because the course of their disease itself was affected but because the disease was detected early and the time between detection and death would be longer. This may account for some of the apparent benefits of screening. However, screening also appears to produce a true increase in survival. (This problem is discussed in a recent ACSH newsletter story.)

The following recommendations for cancer screening reflect consideration by many scientists. The tests suggested are effective, of minimal risk, and of reasonable cost.

BREAST CANCER

Breast cancer will affect approximately one in every ten women. Fortunately, if the cancer is detected early, removal of the tumor will result in a high proportion of cures. Screening for breast cancer has been demonstrated to affect the disease significantly in several well designed studies. In one, using a combination of mammography and physical examination, a 30 percent reduction of mortality after 10 to 15 years was obtained. Screening is a very important aspect of controlling breast cancer.

The simplest method of breast cancer screening is examination of the breasts by hand. It is estimated that this method can detect tumors as small as half an inch in diameter. The advantage of breast self-examination is that if done regularly, the woman will get to know the contour of her own breasts and may then be able to find subtle changes that a physician might not. A physician's exam may be more skilled and might detect changes that have occurred so gradually that the woman herself had not noticed them. Breast examinations usually cost no more than a doctor's office visit and may be included in visits to the doctor for other reasons.

A second method of screening for breast cancer is mammography (a radiographic examination of the breast). Techniques for this have been improving and have about as much exposure to radiation as a chest x-ray. Currently both "screen-film mammography" and "xeromammography" techniques are in use. In both methods the breast is compressed slightly and often two views are taken of each breast. Other than the compression of the breasts, the subject feels nothing. The risks of the procedure relate to the radiation exposure and the potential of increasing the risk of future breast cancer in the person screened. With new techniques and low levels of radiation exposure, the increased risk is estimated to be far less than 1 percent for a lifetime's screening, and calculations have demonstrated that the benefit of mammography far outweighs the risk of the radiation itself. The cost of mammography ranges from $50 to $200, depending on the type of exam and where it is performed.

There are two other methods of testing for breast cancer which are not used widely because they have not been shown to be as valuable as the above techniques. Thermography is a method whereby differences in temperature in the breast are measured on film. A second method is sonography, a technique where sound waves are sent through the breast and their echoes are recorded. Neither method's usefulness for cancer screening has been established.

Many studies, both theoretical and actual, have been done to estimate the best strategy for breast cancer screening. Currently, the following recommendations can be made for a strategy that will reduce mortality, have minimal risk, and be cost effective. For women under forty years of age, a baseline mammogram is recommended. This will detect tumors as well as provide a comparison for future mammograms. Women between the ages of forty and fifty should have mammography every one to two years. The actual interval should be decided upon by the physician. For women fifty and above, annual breast examination and mammography are recommended. How long to continue the exams has not been firmly established, although most physicians will continue the studies through age 65 to 70. Physical examination of the breasts by a physician should be conducted every three years between the ages of twenty and forty. Thereafter, women should have an annual exam. Monthly breast self-examination is also encouraged.

Modifications in the above recommendations should be made by the physician for women at a higher risk of developing breast cancer. This would include women with a mother or sister with breast cancer, or cancer of one breast already diagnosed. Although little or no increased risk has been demonstrated in women with benign proliferative (fibrocystic) breast disease, annual mammography may be instituted at a younger age because of the difficulty in detecting changes in the breast by manual examination.

If a physical exam or mammography detects a new lump or suspicious area, several options are available. If the area is large and easily felt or if it suggests a cyst, a thin needle may be inserted and a small amount of material aspirated into the needle. This can be examined by a pathologist to look for malignant cells. The procedure is almost painless and may be done in a physician's office. Most surgeons, however, prefer to remove the mass, especially if the area is small or difficult to locate. This is minor surgery and may be done in a surgeon's office, day-surgery center, or hospital operating room. Local or general anesthesia may be used depending on the size and depth of the lesion. The material obtained can be frozen and examined immediately by a pathologist or processed and examined more accurately several days later. There are no data that suggest that it is necessary to examine the tissue immediately and proceed to further surgery if it is malignant, although some doctors and patients may choose this option. Only one out of five to ten "suspicious lesions" found by screening will be cancer. The majority will be benign cysts, benign tumors or normal breast tissue. Many women may have several biopsies over their lifetime with none of them being malignant. It is important to realize that women having a negative biopsy still need annual screening, for they are still at risk of developing breast cancer.

COLON AND RECTAL CANCER

Colon and rectal cancer is the second leading cause of cancer deaths in the United States killing an estimated 60,000 people in 1985. Surgery is still the primary treatment for this type of cancer. To obtain a surgical cure, the tumor must be detected at an early stage. As with other cancers, the survival for Stage I (also called Dukes A) colon cancer is much better than the other stages. Early detection of colon and rectal cancer is therefore important and has been shown by several studies to reduce the mortality from these malignancies.

There are several methods of screening for colon and rectal cancer. The simplest is detection of invisible amounts of blood (occult blood) in stool by a test called stool guaiac slide test (formerly fecal occult blood). Tumors of the colon and rectum start in the cells lining the inside wall of the intestine. They then grown out into the passageway of the intestine as well as deeper into the wall itself. Many tumors have a rich supply of blood vessels, and as fecal material scrapes by a tumor, there is often a small amount of bleeding. By testing stool with a special chemical which changes color on contact with tiny quantities of blood, this bleeding can be detected. To accomplish this, a small amount of stool is smeared on a special card which is then brought or mailed to a physician for testing. Three to six samples should be taken over three days. To ensure the accuracy of the test, red meat and vitamins, particularly vitamin C, should not be ingested two days prior to the testing and during the collection. Red meat causes false-positive tests while vitamin C causes false-negative tests. In addition, it is recommended to eat a diet high in fiber prior to and during the testing. The passage of this material across the tumor may stimulate a tiny amount of bleeding and thus help detect the tumor. It will not affect the normal lining of the intestine.

The cost of this test is about five dollars, and kits are available from a pharmacy without a prescription. Often physicians will do the test without charge as part of an office visit or follow-up. Only between one in fifteen or one in twenty persons with positive tests will actually have colon or rectal cancer. This is because many other conditions of the colon or rectum, most of which are not serious, can cause a positive test. Therefore, individuals having a positive test should receive further tests as described below.

Another simple test for colon or rectal cancer is the digital exam in which the physician inserts a gloved, lubricated finger into the rectum to feel for abnormalities. While the test is uncomfortable, it poses no risk to the individual and is also useful in looking for cancer of the prostate. If an abnormality such as a mass is found, it must be evaluated further.

The best way to look for cancer of the colon or rectum is to actually visualize their surface. There are two methods for doing this, the first utilizing a rigid instrument called a proctoscope. This is a tube about three-quarters of an inch in diameter and eleven inches long. On the outer end is placed a light source through which the physician can look. The patient is positioned on a table and using lubricant, the tube is introduced into the rectum and advanced under visual guidance into the sigmoid colon (the lowest part of the colon). If the patient has received sufficient preparation, the doctor can see the lining of the rectum and sigmoid colon very well. Should a suspicious lesion be visualized, it is possible to take a biopsy of the lesion while the proctoscope is in place. The procedure is performed in a physician's office and is uncomfortable for the patient.

The main risk of the procedure is breaking through the lining of the intestine. This is very rare, occurring much less than one in a thousand procedures. Its main disadvantage is that it can only visualize part of the colon. To view a greater portion of the colon, a longer, flexible device called a flexible sigmoidoscope or colonoscope must be used.

A flexible sigmoidoscope is a rubber-like tube slightly smaller in diameter than a proctoscope. It uses a fiberoptic light source in which light is carried down the fibers as well as back, enabling the user to see around the bends in the tube as it is passed through the rectum into the colon. Lengths of the tube vary, but it is usually about twice as long as a proctoscope. A colonoscope is a similar device but much longer. Although more difficult to use, it is more effective in detecting cancer since it visualizes the entire colon. These scopes also have attachments to biopsy a suspicious lesion if found. A flexible sigmoidoscope is similar in discomfort to a rigid proctoscope.

Colonoscopy is a more involved procedure and patients are usually given medicine intravenously to help them relax. For this reason, colonoscopy is not suitable for general screening. A sigmoidoscopy carries essentially the same risk as a proctoscopy, whereas a colonoscopy has a greater risk of perforation. It is still, however, a very safe procedure. The cost of a proctoscopy is about $50, sigmoidoscopy is more expensive and a colonoscopy will cost several hundred dollars.

Another procedure which may detect colon cancer is a barium enema x-ray. Barium, a substance which can be seen by x-ray, is passed into the colon with an enema. The patient is rotated in various positions and a radiologist watches with a fluoroscope while the barium coats the wall of the intestine. In this way, an outline of the wall can be obtained and any irregularities noted. This test is less useful in detecting colon cancers because small lesions may be missed and if a lesion is identified, a sigmoidoscopy or colonoscopy will be necessary anyway to biopsy the lesion. It may be useful in patients who cannot tolerate a sigmoidoscopy.

The most reasonable and effective screening method for colon cancer is for individuals over fifty years of age to have a yearly test for occult blood and a flexible sigmoidoscopy every three years. An alternative is to have proctoscopy every year in place of the sigmoidoscopy. Individuals with a history of colonic polyps or previous colon cancer should have more frequent tests as recommended by their physician. It is estimated that screening in this manner could reduce the mortality from colon and rectal cancer up to 40 percent.

As mentioned above, if a person has a positive test for occult blood, further testing is necessary. This usually involves a combination of proctoscopy and a barium enema or a colonoscopy. Most of the time the cause of bleeding will be benign, such as diverticulosis or hemorrhoids. If no abnormalities are found, the positive test may be attributed to bleeding higher up in the digestive tract. Depending on the individual circumstances, the physician may decide that further tests are necessary.

Occasionally, proctoscopy, sigmoidoscopy, colonoscopy, or a barium enema will reveal a colonic polyp. A polyp is a growth of tissue from the wall of the intestine which often resembles a mushroom. Polyps range in size from almost too small to see to up to several inches in diameter. They are usually benign growths like moles on the skin but can become malignant. The larger polyps and certain shapes of polyps are more likely to be malignant. Polyps are removed when they are seen. (Occasionally very small polyps may be left in place and followed by repeat examinations.) The tissue is then processed and examined by a pathologist to determine if it is malignant. No treatment other than repeat examinations is necessary in patients with benign polyps. In patients with a diagnosis of cancer, further treatment (surgery) is usually necessary. The exact type of treatment is based upon the extent to which the tumor has spread. Hopefully, screening will detect polyps before they become malignant or when they are at a very early stage of malignancy. Very rarely, screening will detect a large growth in the colon or rectum. In this case, a biopsy is taken and further treatment planned according to the results of the biopsy and extent of the tumor.

Frequent Aspirin Use May Reduce Risk of Several Fatal Digestive Tract Cancers

In the 1990s research began to surface suggesting that people who regularly use aspirin may have a lower risk of fatal cancers of the esophagus, stomach, and rectum, as well as colon.

In an American Cancer Society study, death rates from all four digestive tract cancers were approximately 40 percent lower among men and women who used aspirin 16 times per month or more for at least one year compared to those who used no aspirin. The trend of decreasing risk with more frequent aspirin use was strongest among persons who had used aspirin for 10 years or more. In contrast, death rates from other cancers were not associated with aspirin use.

There is evidence that aspirin may prevent cancer by inhibiting cell proliferation, tumor growth, tumor promotion, and metastases, and enhance immune responses.

There is, at this time, currently insufficient information to recommend aspirin to prevent cancer. This is a new research area, and we need results from other studies and especially from clinical trials before we can make such a widespread recommendation. Also, we have to consider that aspirin, although relatively innocuous to most people, can cause serious adverse reactions in some.

Screening Our Children for Cancer

Cancer is the most common cause of death due to disease in children over the age of one year. Malignant diseases occur in about 10 per 100,000 children per year and account for approximately 4,000 deaths annually. While leukemias and lymphomas constitute about 40 percent of pediatric malignant diseases, solid tumors make up the remaining 60 percent.

The most common solid tumor of infancy and early childhood is neuroblastoma. This tumor accounts for 50 percent of all cancers encountered in the neonate and approximately 30 percent of malignant conditions diagnosed in the first year of life. A highly aggressive cancer of the peripheral nervous system, this disease is characterized by painful tumor masses in areas such as the abdomen, along the spine, on the skull, or behind the eye.

Unfortunately, cancer in most kids with neuroblastoma is diagnosed only after it has spread throughout the body. Disseminated disease will be found in 70 percent of children more than one-year-old and in 50 percent of those less than one year.

A child with neuroblastoma can probably be saved if his or her tumor has been detected earlier. If diagnosed before the tumor becomes clinically obvious, simple surgical removal can assure the child a greater than 95 percent cure rate. Neuroblastoma is, in fact, the only childhood tumor for which early detection is feasible. Neuroblastoma produces chemicals called catecholamines that are excreted in the urine. The presence of these chemicals can be detected with a simple urine test. Such a screening test performed at the age of six months may very possibly save a child's life.

Neuroblastoma has an estimated incidence of 1:6,000 to 1:10,000 meaning that it is more common than at least three other diseases that are routinely and mandatorily screened for by most states.

Mass screening of newborn infants for metabolic diseases was made possible in the 1960s with the discovery of a simple test for a disorder known as phenylketonuria (PKU). This screening test is performed on a small sample of blood obtained on filter paper by sticking the baby's heel. Advances in assay techniques have allowed a variety of other disorders to be identified. Each state legislates the specific diseases to be screened and the mechanics of the screening and follow-up process. The following table offers an example of the comparative incidences of diseases mandatorily screened and paid for by almost every state.

Table 12.1
Mandatory Newborn Screening
Comparative Incidence Data

Disease	Incidence
Galactosemia	1:76,000
PKU	1:33,000
Congenital Adrenal Hyperplasia	1:15,000
Hypothyroidism	1: 3,400
Hemoglobinopathies	1: 500

Japan has had regional mass screening programs to detect neuroblastoma since 1972 and has had a mandatory nationwide mass screening program since 1985. The incidence of this tumor is comparable in Japan, the United States and the United Kingdom. In a recent study a comparison of the survival rates of all neuroblastoma patients in Japan increased from 17 percent before screening to 71 percent after the onset of screening. This data included all children. Of the six-month-old infants detected, 96 percent were cured. It is very important to note that, of the six-month-old infants diagnosed, more than 90 percent had absolutely no symptoms.

Dr. Joanne Ater, a pediatric cancer specialist at Houston's M.D. Anderson Career Center, has developed a Texas-based study program to test the effectiveness of mass screening for neuroblastoma in the U.S. This monumental neuroblastoma study will screen 300,000 infants born in Texas during 1992 and 1993. Treatment results of children diagnosed from the pilot study will be pooled, then compared with the outcome of patients not screened, in order to document the impact of the program. Dr. Ater's group is utilizing a newer and less costly technique than that used by the Japanese researchers. This ELISA method uses monoclonal antibodies to the urinary catecholamines and should prove more specific and more sensitive than the high-performance liquid chromatography (HPLC) techniques used in the Japanese program. Dr. Ater's group has designed a very simple mail-out kit to collect urine samples. This kit contains a bilingual information brochure, an informed consent and data sheet, a piece of filter paper in a plastic specimen bag and a self-addressed envelope in which to return the sample. Parents need only collect the urine on the filter paper, either directly or by application to a wet diaper, allow the sample to dry, then mail it in. Adequate attention has been given in the information brochure to the possibility of needing a repeat sample. Those who test positive can be referred to M.D. Anderson for complete evaluation or may be evaluated by any of a regional network of cooperating pediatric oncologists.

Unfortunately, it's probably too late for Josh. But it's not too late for the generations to come. If diagnosed early enough, neuroblastoma is greater than 95 percent curable with one simple surgery. The time to screen for this deadly childhood cancer has arrived. I'm sure Dr. Ater's extraordinary study will confirm the Japanese studies. Every state in the U.S. needs to consider adding this simple yet invaluable screening test to its neonatal screening program.

Screening for Cervical Cancer

The Papanicolau (Pap) smear, introduced in 1943, remains the mainstay of cervical cancer screening around the world.

The test involves scraping cell samples from the outer portion of the cervix (the lower part of the uterus) and the endocervical canal (inside the cervical opening).

This test was designed as a cost effective way to evaluate large numbers of people reliably and reproducibly. However, a routine Pap smear will miss up to ten percent of cervical carcinomas because of errors made while acquiring the sample, pathological misinterpretation at the laboratory or the inability to detect certain types of pathology.

While there is a general consensus that appropriate evaluation can diagnose early cell changes and lead to definitive treatment of precancerous stages, there is little agreement about what "appropriate evaluation" means. The American College of Obstetricians and Gynecologists (ACOG) recommends that a Pap smear be done for all women by the age of 18 or when sexually active, whichever comes first. Follow-up evaluation should be done annually in women with multiple sexual partners. The ACOG also recommends that those in long-term relationships who have had three negative annual Pap smears in a row may be screened less often.

Cervical carcinoma remains one of the most curable forms of gynecologic cancer, especially if diagnosed early. In general, cure rates using either radiotherapy or surgery in early cancers of the cervix range from 85 to 95 percent. Nevertheless, the incidence remains high for a carcinoma thought to be "completely preventable." As a result, screening, in order to prevent a precancerous stage from developing further, takes on a greater importance. Regular Pap smears and follow-up, especially in women who have HPV or multiple sex partners, is the most effective way to prevent cervical cancer.

Actions That May Not (But Could) Prevent Cancer: What They Don't Tell You About Prostate Cancer

Roger, an insurance executive, was fifty-four when first diagnosed as having prostate cancer. He underwent radical prostatectomy soon after diagnosis. Two years later his Prostate-Specific Antigen (PSA) reading was again elevated, and he underwent radiation therapy.

> I had never felt sick a day of my life. Just over two years ago I went in feeling fine for my annual physical, and I came out half a man.
>
> The year before, my internist had noticed a little nodule on my prostate and ordered a biopsy, which took little bits from all over the gland for microscopic inspection. It came up negative. I forgot about the whole thing and thought that was that. But a year later the nodule was still there, and the urologist did a PSA. It was 15 or 16, and that's pretty high. The urologist did a sonogram of the suspicious area and took a biopsy. This time it turned out to be positive. He immediately recommended surgery.
>
> I shopped around for other advice—four different doctors, although in retrospect I probably should have gotten more variety of opinion, as all four were surgeons, and from the same hospital. They all said the same thing: You are too young not to take immediate action. That meant removal of the prostate gland.
>
> I was in the hospital for two weeks, and it was hardly routine: I developed a blood clot that could have been life-threatening, and they put me on a blood-thinner for months after the operation. But at least, I thought, the nightmare was over. The word from the doctors was that, assuming there was no other sign of cancer and the tumor was limited

to the gland, I was home free. I could put it in a little jar on the mantel and I would be golden. I sincerely believed that after the radical I was out of the woods.

But two years later, during another routine physical, my internist noted casually that my PSA was up to 15 again. He didn't seem upset, so initially I was not. But that night I saw Senator Dole on television discussing the fact that he has an elevated PSA of four, and I was alarmed for myself—also puzzled, wondering why I had a PSA reading at all when I had no prostate gland. [An elevated PSA reading after surgery may be evidence that the cancer has spread.]

I found myself right back in the medical maze, with bone and CAT scans, and an eventual diagnosis that "maybe" there were some lurking cancer cells in what they call the "prostate bed." I was told that cobalt radiation was the answer. Again, I had no symptoms. The radiation was to kill the cancer cells that might be there. The psychological as well as the physical symptoms of that treatment were overwhelming for me, but what choice did I have?

Now I'm playing the waiting game again, waiting three months to get another PSA. Waiting for some magic number that will determine the rest of my life.

I was told, when first considering surgery, that I faced a 50-50 chance of impotence and incontinence. The potential loss of sexual ability was extremely important to me. My wife and I pressed this point with my doctors, many of whom seemed annoyed by my questions and perplexed that sex was important to me when they were saying that my life was in danger. "I'm going to save your life, Roger," one physician said. "I don't want to talk about the ancillary matters." But for me these ancillary matters were just as important as prostate cancer. I might not want to live if

I were sexually incapacitated.

One surgeon thought he had the answer to calm my concerns: He recommended that I interview a patient on whom he had just performed a prostatectomy. I did so, only to learn from this 65year-old man that he had no concerns whatever about sexual dysfunction because he and his wife had "given that up" years ago. Now he just wanted to "live long enough to play some good golf." That was not my view, and I would have been appreciative if the physicians counseling us had understood the importance of quality of life as well as length of life. (The 65-year-old man later asked our mutual doctor why he had sent a "sex maniac" to interview him.)

Physicians seem to want to put a pretty face on everything, withholding important information, preferring to give you bad news a little bit at a time. I would have preferred it all up front. If I had known the full implications of the temporary incontinence I faced, I would have dealt with it much more effectively. But I was not informed.

—*Priorities* (Fall 1992)

In the checkup department, men over age fifty have recently been urged to have regular examinations for prostate cancer, including a new test called the Prostate-Specific Antigen test, or PSA. In the words of a physician writing in *Priorities* (Fall 1992, pp. 27–32), a quarterly magazine that I publish:

The PSA should be to cancer of the prostate what the Pap smear is to cancer of the uterus and cervix, and what mammography is to breast cancer. Men should be trading their PSA numbers right along with their cholesterol scores—at the office, in the spa, playing golf, wherever men gather.

It all sounded so simple: Find the cancer early, cut it out, and you're home free. Since publishing that well-meaning article, however, I have learned that it presented only a fraction of the story and that it offered far-reaching advice that would not necessarily deliver the promised results. Here, to set the record straight, is the disturbing truth about the detection and treatment of prostate cancer, and about the highly touted PSA.

The prostate is a walnut-size gland at the base of the bladder, surrounding the urethra. It weighs only about 20 grams and is composed of gland, muscle, vascular, and fibrous tissue. The prostate gland is one of three structures that generate seminal fluid, which mixes with sperm just before ejaculation.

Many people have only the foggiest idea of what the prostate is or does. (In a 1990 article, *Esquire* referred several times to the "prostrate" gland.) It deserves more attention: The prostate can be a source of great discomfort (enlargement is common in older men), and it can be the site of a life-threatening condition. This year, more than 132,000 American men will be diagnosed as having prostate cancer, and 34,000 will die of it; the only types of cancer that kill more American men are lung and colon cancer. The number of new cases has increased in the past two decades, in part because of better detection, but the death rate has also increased slightly.

The disease has taken on some familiar faces in the news recently: Senators Robert Dole of Kansas and Alan Cranston of California; Roone Arledge, president of ABC; and Steven Ross, the chief executive of Time Warner, are among those who have said publicly that they have prostate cancer. Frank Zappa, the rock musician, and Joseph Papp, the producer, recently died of it.

Still, there has been little discussion of the disease among either patients or doctors. A review of the past three years of major medical journals, including *The New England Journal of Medicine, Lancet, The Journal of the American Medical Association,* and *Science,* reveals only a handful of articles on this killer disease, versus an overwhelming number of research articles on such topics as AIDS, breast cancer, and colon cancer.

Perhaps acknowledging that prostate cancer has been the victim of neglect, the National Cancer Institute doubled the amount of money spent for research on the disease, from $14 million in 1991 to $28 million this year. Still, compare that with the $133 million spent on research into breast cancer, or the $83 million spent on lung cancer.

To understand the problem surrounding the detection and treatment of prostate cancer, it is essential to recognize that this type of cancer in some form is extremely common, particularly as men age, but that it often grows slowly, and in many cases is not life-threatening. Scientists currently estimate that 11 million American men have prostate cancer in some form, although only a fraction have been diagnosed. Signs of the disease are found during the autopsies of almost all men ninety or over who have died of other causes; the figure is 41 percent in men aged forty to forty-nine, and 22 percent in men between thirty and thirty-nine. In other words, there is a large discrepancy between the number of men who have some form of prostate cancer and the number of men who show signs of the disease. This fact is critical when it comes to evaluating the need for mass screening and the options for treatment.

The "gold standard" of prostate detection has long been

the digital rectal examination (DRE), hailed as "easy to perform" and "inexpensive," but rejected by many men. Even though the test can usually be done quickly, with little discomfort, some men will not submit to a rectal exam unless they are having severe problems, usually related to urination. Furthermore, the DRE is short on sensitivity: thirty percent to 60 percent of men with prostate cancer have tumors that the examining physician cannot feel. In fact, most men with early prostate cancer—presumably the stage at which a cure is most likely—have no symptoms at all.

On the reasonable assumption that more men could be saved if we could detect cancer before it spread beyond the gland, researchers looked for new screening techniques to replace or supplement the DRE. A number of new techniques now exist, including ultrasonography. But the method that has made headlines for "new and improved screening for prostate cancer" is the PSA, a blood test that measures a substance secreted only by the prostatic epithelial cells. The immediate advantages of the PSA are that it is objective, quantifiable, and more comfortable than the DRE. But even its most enthusiastic proponents acknowledge that the PSA has limitations: Its results include both false negatives and false positives. A man can have prostate cancer, even in an advanced stage, and still have a normal PSA reading. Or an enlarged but not cancerous prostate can elevate the PSA.

Many doctors are now embracing the PSA as warmly as gynecologists do the Pap smear for early detection of cervical cancer. But certain facts remain unclear:

An unknown number of prostate cancers detected by any means, including the PSA, may be "dormant," meaning that they will never progress to life-threatening disease. Proponents disagree, arguing that the PSA picks up only those cancers that are clinically important, but the question is definitely still open for debate.

Even with the addition of the PSA to the screening scene, depressing statistics characterize today's diagnosis: For every 1,000 men diagnosed as having prostate cancer, 333 will be classified as "noncurable" because the malignancy has spread to surrounding tissues; the remaining men will be categorized as "curable" on the assumption that the disease is gland-limited, and will be urged to undergo treatment, which is almost always radical prostatectomy, the removal of the prostate gland. (This is the preferred treatment in the United States, but not in Western Europe, where radiation therapy is more in vogue.)

More than half of the 667 "curable" patients, within a year or two of the operation to remove the prostate (and sometimes during the operation itself), are found to be "noncurable" after all, meaning that metastasis (spread) of the cancer has already occurred.

In other words, even when the PSA is used in conjunction with other tests, it appears that two-thirds of patients who develop clinically detectable prostate cancer are already beyond the point where a cure is possible—"cure" being defined here as the complete removal of a gland to which cancer was completely confined. There is little or nothing to be gained by removing the prostate in patients whose cancer has already spread; it's extremely difficult to remove cancer from the surrounding tissues, or to control it, and experts do not advocate the "debulking" of tumors that cannot be removed completely.

But even if the PSA catches only a tiny percentage of cancers, doesn't the saving of those few lives justify screening "just in case," especially as the test is simple and almost painless? This would be a worthy argument if the PSA had no dangers associated with it. Unfortunately, though the test itself is quick and harmless, the possible consequences are not.

Advocates, say critics of the test, ignore the potential harm of diagnosing cancers that would not shorten lives. First of all, any major surgery carries a certain amount of risk; the death rate associated with prostatectomy is 1 percent to 2 percent. If 30 percent of the 25 million screened men over fifty had cancer detected and subsequently excised in surgery (not an unreasonable estimate, considering the autopsy figures cited earlier), a 1 percent mortality rate would mean 75,000 deaths—45,000 more than would be expected from the cancer itself.

Second, prostatectomy carries a fairly high risk of causing impotence, incontinence, or both, especially in older men.

Third, the test is relatively expensive—$85 or more. "Even if Medicare would offer reimbursement, the test cost is prohibitive," says Dr. William R. Fair, chief of urology at the Memorial Sloan-Kettering Cancer Center in New York City. He points out that screening 28 million American men over fifty could cost $2.4 billion, "$400 million more than the National Cancer Institute's entire budget."

Fourth, even men who are correctly diagnosed as having cancer may not benefit from surgery. In some men the cancer will be found to have already spread, making surgery worthless, and in some, particularly older men, the cancer would never have progressed to the life-threatening stage, making surgery unnecessary.

In the words of Dr. Frank Hinman, Jr., of the department of urology at the University of California School of Medicine in San Francisco, "The cumulative harmful effects of screening many men may outweigh the benefits of earlier diagnosis of a few."

A barnyard analogy has been used to shed light on the problem. Suppose you wanted to build a fence to keep three kinds of animals—turtles, birds, and rabbits—on your property. The birds would soon be gone, flying over the fence to parts unknown. The turtles would plod around slowly, but none would reach the edge of the property. The rabbits would hop around, and eventually, unless you stopped them, they would clear the fence and escape. In other words, the fence would be effective only for the rabbits. The turtles don't need it, and the birds would ignore it.

If we apply this analogy to clinical prostate cancer, the birds are men who are beyond cure, because their malignancies have metastasized. To treat these men with surgery not only would fail to lead to a cure, it would, as Hinman says, "set up a sequence of diagnostic steps and treatment programs that might seriously interfere with the quality of life." These patients can benefit only from palliative care— that is, nonsurgical assistance to make them more comfortable and possibly extend their lives. But there are no figures on how long palliative care can extend life, because no follow-up studies have been done. We should also realize that screening would make thousands of men aware that they have an incurable disease, with no effective options for treatment, long before any problems would otherwise surface. Since nothing could be done, many would probably prefer not to know.

The turtles are patients with low-grade, nonaggressive, non-lifethreatening prostate cancers. These men do not need screening or treatment. To find these cancers would cause anxiety and grief, and probably some very undesirable consequences should surgery be recommended. The turtles should be left to wander aimlessly and harmlessly. Patients in the third group, the rabbits, are the only ones who stand to benefit from screening.

Treating all the men diagnosed as having prostate cancer, therefore, would mean saving the lives of a third of them, at most, at the cost of some degree of unnecessary incapacitation in twice as many others.

The emerging medical consensus, which hasn't quite made it to the popular press, is that what we need is not more screening, but methods of determining which of the prostate-confined cancers are "real" and would benefit from surgery, and which of them are harmless and should be let alone. Further, we need a way of determining, before surgery, which men with cancers that are initially diagnosed as "curable"— a group comprising two thirds of all patients—are really "birds," who have nothing to gain from treatment.

Dr. Willet F. Whitmore, Jr., the recently retired head of the department of urology at Sloan-Kettering Cancer Center in New York, has phrased the problem another way: "Is cure possible in those for whom it is necessary, and is cure necessary in those for whom it is possible?" (In the medical literature this is known as "Whitmore's question.")

Dr. Gerald Chodak, director of urologic oncology at the University of Chicago Pritzker School of Medicine, argues that the following criteria must be satisfied to justify mass screening of men for prostate cancer. First, the means of early detection of cancers should be improved. Second, there must be evidence that screened men survive longer than unscreened men. Third, there must be evidence that the death rate from prostate cancer has decreased. None of these criteria, says Dr. Chodak, has so far been met. "We must conclude," he says, "that currently there is no scientific proof that screening is justified." The Centers for Disease Control recently agreed: "The value of mass screening for prostate cancer . . . is unclear."

Dr. Fair of Sloan-Kettering is even more skeptical. "PSA could also stand for Priority Seems Awry," he says. "We don't have any evidence that early detection leads to increased survival, and we don't have the faintest clue of how to distinguish indolent from aggressive prostate cancers."

"The PSA is a useful tool in following patients with known prostate cancer, but it is still not a useful tool for screening," says Dr. Michael P. O'Leary of New England Medical Center in Boston. "It is not sensitive or specific enough." This is also the position of The National Cancer Institute, which still recommends that a rectal exam "be part of a regular checkup for all men over 40, but does not recommend that the PSA be used for diagnosis.

But some physicians, such as Dr. William J. Catalona of the Washington University School of Medicine in St. Louis, remain enthusiastic about mass screening with the PSA and other techniques. "It is very conceivable," he writes, "that using [these techniques], the statistics in prostate cancer could be dramatically altered. Instead of seven out of 10 cancers being advanced at the time of diagnosis, we could flip that and seven out of 10 could be in the early stage."

Dr. Ruben F. Gittes of the Scripps Clinic and Research Foundation in La Jolla, California, agrees unequivocally. "I think it is just as important as having a cholesterol test," he says.

Finally, there are those doctors who support prostate testing but acknowledge that its value has yet to be proved.

"This issue has never been studied, and no one has ever shown that an early diagnosis of prostate cancer does not prolong survival," says Dr. Patrick Walsh of Johns Hopkins Hospital (arguing, in effect, that the test is innocent until proved guilty).

"I think urologists should continue to practice and encourage periodic examination of the prostate in men older than 50 years," says Dr. Paul H. Lange of the department of urologic surgery at the University of Washington School of Medicine in Seattle.

> If the purpose of the examination is to detect as many "clinical" cancers as possible, today such an examination should include the PSA. We must also continue to admit that this approach is controversial. I believe that aggressive early diagnosis and treatment of prostate cancer are beneficial, but we must prove it.

When deciding whether you should undergo screening for prostate cancer, there are a number of things to consider. First of all, though it seems clear that from a societal point of view mass screening is not currently justified, there may also be individual considerations, such as a family history of prostate cancer. For men in this category, regular screening may catch what are likely to develop into life-threatening cancers if left untreated.

Even Dr. Fair, hardly an advocate of PSA testing, agrees that the test has its uses.

> I view the PSA in much the same way as the serum cholesterol or a proctoscopy. I do not believe that it should be one of our national health priorities to do a PSA on

every man over the age of 50. However, in men who want the most complete, thorough evaluation, a digital rectal examination and a PSA would be appropriate.

Your age should be a consideration. Some physicians argue that testing before age fifty is not necessary or cost-effective because the frequency of clinically detectable cancers is so low, and that tests after the age of seventy are not needed because of the low likelihood that prostate cancer will be a life-threatening condition in men of that age.

But suppose that you have been screened, and the test comes up positive. What should you do if you are diagnosed as having prostate cancer? I recommended the following:

Seek advice not only from your potential surgeon, but from "disinterested parties" as well. This is not to suggest that your surgeon necessarily has a mercenary interest in getting you into the operating room, but worries about litigation, and the basic human desire to try to help, may make him more prone to suggest treatment than to recommend doing nothing. And, after all, cutting is what he was trained to do. Ideally, a "tumor board" made up of a number of specialists should evaluate your case.

Understand that current medical science cannot predict what any specific tumor will do in the future.

Consider treatment other than surgery. Speak with a radiation oncologist about radiation therapy, and with a urologist about hormone therapy. Also, be aware that the risk of long-term impotence and incontinence stemming from radiation or hormone therapy may be similar to those associated with surgery.

Take an extremely active role in the decision. Read the medical literature: Go to a medical library and look up prostate cancer in the Index Medicus. Disregard any literature that is older than two or three years.

"It is essential that the patient take on an aggressive, active role in deciding what kind of treatment to have," says Dr. Barrie R. Cassileth, a consulting professor at the medical centers of Duke University and the University of North Carolina. "If they know only what their urologist tells them, for example, they are more likely to have surgery."

Ask for information on the "staging" of the cancer. Cancers are usually given a rating from A to D; A and B mean that the cancer may or may not have spread beyond the gland, and C and D mean that it probably has. The stage is very important in deciding on a type of treatment. Some men with stage A prostate cancer, in the opinion of some urologists, need not be treated at all.

Involve your wife in the decision. Dr. Chodak of the University of Chicago emphasizes this: "The women have a lot to deal with. Impotence and incontinence affect their lives as well."

Ask about the options for treatment, and about the consequences of doing nothing.

The option of doing nothing for early prostate cancer received much publicity in April 1992, when a Swedish research team, writing in *The Journal of the American Medical Association,* concluded that men with early prostate cancer who are not treated for their disease have an excellent survival rate, rivaling that of patients who receive aggressive therapy. For a substantial group of these patients, primarily those in their seventies, doing nothing proved to be as good as or better than surgery or radiation therapy. Approximately 12 percent of both the treated and untreated men in this study died of prostate cancer within ten years of the diagnosis.

Some doctors applauded this research for highlighting the scientific ignorance about the best way to approach prostate cancer. But advocates of screening condemned the study, claiming that it would lull men into believing that prostate cancer was a relatively benign condition. "I think it could absolutely misdirect people," says Dr. Walsh of Johns Hopkins. "This could be very harmful. That the *Journal of the American Medical Association* would accept a paper like this absolutely shocks me."

Take your age into account. Some physicians believe that not doing anything may be the best option for men over seventy. Patients under sixty, whose prostates are bathed in high doses of natural testosterone (which promotes tumor growth), may be more at risk of an aggressive progression of the cancer. It is Dr. Fair's opinion that radical prostatectomy should not be considered for any man whose life expectancy is less than ten years.

Understand the consequences of whatever option you choose, whether it be surgery, radiation, hormone therapy, or doing nothing. There is much talk now about a greatly diminished frequency of impotence and incontinence after radical prostatectomy. Just a few years ago, the likelihood of impotence was nearly 100 percent. Physicians now say that new "nerve-sparing" techniques have reduced this probability tremendously.

Even so, the chance of side effects, particularly impotence, remains high—perhaps more than 40 percent, especially in patients over the age of sixty. The National Cancer Institute stated several years ago that patients should be provided with information on "probability of cure, mortality, complications, and other side effects of radical prostatectomy and radiation therapy; risk of impotence and incontinence for either treatment; psychosocial consequences of either choice; [and] economic consequences of each form of treatment."

Ask your doctor this question: If I proceed with surgery, is there a significant chance that we will later find that the cancer had already spread—in which case I will have had a useless procedure that may have caused physical dysfunction? The honest answer here is yes. The odds of this no-win situation are something you will want to discuss with your physician.

A recent article on prostate cancer in *Science* magazine stated: "Given a choice between impotence or death from disseminated cancer, most people would choose impotence." That may well be true. But, as we have seen, the situation is not that simple. There are probably quite a few men who would choose eight to ten more years of relatively normal life over a non-guaranteed operation with a high risk of dysfunction.

In other words, when deciding whether to undergo treatment for prostate cancer, consider the quality of life, not just the extension of life. In the words of Dr. Whitmore of Sloan-Kettering Cancer Center, "quality survival" is a legitimate alternative to "cure" in selected patients with prostatic cancer.

Consider participating in a clinical trial of a new treatment for prostate cancer. Call the national Cancer Institute (1-800-4-CANCER) and request the publication *What are Clinical Trials All About?*

Although it is impossible at this point to make specific recommendations, either for individuals or for society, on the desirability of screening or the "correct" option for dealing with what appears to be gland-limited prostate cancer, a review of the current literature leads one to the conclusion that the money being spent on mass screening for prostate cancer might be spent in much better ways, such as:

- looking for means of distinguishing among latent prostate cancer, potentially life-threatening but curable cancer, and incurable cancer. With such techniques, massive screening would make more sense; the growing proportion of men diagnosed with gland-limited cancer could be assured that treatment would indeed save their lives, and men with dormant cancers or cancers that had already metastasized would be spared unnecessary surgery and its side effects. "The great need at present," Hinman writes, "is not to find more cancers but to be able to detect only those that will be harmful."

- seeking additional nonsurgical treatments for prostate cancer.

- learning why some men (particularly black Americans) are more at risk of developing prostate cancer, in order to institute programs that can prevent the disease in the first place.

- testing promising new drugs that might prevent the clinical onset of prostate cancer in high-risk men.

Medical science is currently engaged in a desperate attempt to find cancers early, using techniques that lead us to "cure" cancers that pose no threat and to treat cancers that are beyond help. There are, as we have seen, plenty of alternatives worth considering—alternatives to screening, alternatives to surgery or other treatment, and certainly alternative ways to spend the money now being used for a test that raises many more questions than it answers.

References

Chapter 1: Establishing the Causes of Human Cancer

*American Council on Science and Health. 1991. *From Mice to Men: The Benefits and Limitations of Animal Testing in Predicting Human Cancer Risk.* New York.

Ames, B., and L. Gold. 1991. Endogenous mutagens and the causes of aging and cancer. *Mut. Res.* 250: 3-16.

Cutler, R. G. 1991. Human longevity and aging: possible role of reactive oxygen species. *Ann. N.Y. Acad. Sciences* 62: 1-20.

Doll, R. 1991. Progress against cancer: an epidemiologic assessment. The 1991 John C. Cassel Memorial Lecture. *American Journal of Epidemiology* 134: 675-88.

———. 1992. Are we winning the war against cancer? A review in memory of Keith Durrant. *Clinical Oncology* 4: 257-66.

Evans, P. H., A. K. Champbell, E. Yano, et al. 1989. Environmental cancer, phagocytic oxidant stress and nutritional interactions. *Bibl. Nutr. Dieta.* (Basel: Karger) 43: 313-26.

---

*Indicates reading material that is readily accessible to the average lay person.

375

Martin, G. 1991. Genetic and environmental modulation of chromosomal stability: their role in aging and oncogenesis. *Ann. N.Y. Acad. Sci.* 621: 401–417.

Weitzman, S. A., and L. I. Gordon. 1990. Inflammation and cancer: Role of phagocyte-generated oxidants in carcinogenesis. *Blood* 76: 655–63.

Whittemore, A. S. 1989. Cancer risk assessment and prevention: Where do we stand? *Environmental Health Perspectives* 81: 95–101.

Chapter 2: A Cancer Epidemic?

*American Cancer Society. *Cancer Facts and Figures—1994.*

Bailar III, J. C., and E. M. Smith. 1986. Progress against cancer? *The New England Journal of Medicine* 314: 1226–32.

Baquet, C. R., et al. March 1986. *Cancer among blacks and other minorities: Statistical profiles.* NIH Publication No. 86–2785. Bethesda, Md.: National Cancer Institute.

*Boring, C. C., T. S. Squires, and T. Tong. 1993. Cancer Statistics 1993. *CA: A Cancer Journal for Clinicians* 43: 7–26.

Henderson, B. E., R. K. Ross, and M. C. Pike. 1991. Toward the primary prevention of cancer. *Science* 254: 1131–37.

Miller, B. A., L. A. G. Reis, B. F., Hankey, et al., eds. 1992. *Cancer Statistics Review: 1973–1989.* NIH Pub. No. 92–2789. Bethesda, Md.: National Cancer Institute.

Sondik, E. J. et al. March 1986. *1985 Annual Cancer Statistics Review.* NIH Publication No. 86–2789. Bethesda, Md.: National Cancer Institute.

Tomatis, L., et al. 1990. *Cancer: Causes, Occurrence and Control.* IARC Scientific Publication No. 100. World Health Organization, International Agency for Research on Cancer.

Chapter 3: Tobacco

*American Council on Science and Health. 1993. *Smoking or Health: It's Your Choice.* New York.

*Lane, S. M. 1993. *Marketing Cigarettes to Kids: A Consumer Guide to the Harmful Tactics of Tobacco Companies.* New York: American Council on Science and Health.

*Whelan, E. M. *The Smoking Gun* (forthcoming).

Chapter 4: Alcohol

*American Council on Science and Health. 1993. *Does Moderate Alcohol Consumption Prolong Life?* New York.

Christen, J. A., and A. G. Christen. 1991. Understanding addiction. *J. Indiana Dent. Assn.* 70: 16–19.

Naccarato, R., and F. Farinati. 1991. Hepatocellular carcinoma, alcohol, and cirrhosis: Facts and hypotheses. *Digestive Diseases and Sciences* 36: 1137–42.

Plant, M. L. 1992. Alcohol and breast cancer: A review. *The International Journal of the Addictions* 27: 107–138.

Tyun, A. J. 1991. Aetiology of head and neck cancer: Tobacco, alcohol and diet. In *Bearing of Basic Research on Clinical Otolaryngology,* ed. C. R. Pfaltz, W. Arnold, and O. Kleinsasser. Basel: Karger. *Adv. Otorhinolaryngol.* 46: 98–106.

Chapter 5: Sunlight

*American Academy of Dermatology:
   Melanoma/Skin Cancer
   The Sun and Your Skin
   Sun Protection for Your Children

Moles
American Cancer Society
   Facts on Skin Cancer
   Fry Now, Pay Later
   What You Should Know About Melanoma
*American Council on Science and Health. 1986. *Malignant Melanoma of the Skin: An Increasingly Common Cancer.* New York.
*The Skin Cancer Foundation. *Types and Descriptions of Skin Cancers.*

Chapter 6: Radiation: Managing Technology Safely

*American Council on Science and Health. 1993. *Health Effects of Low-Level Radiation.* New York.

Christian Science Monitor, May 8, 1992.

*Cobb, E. C. April 1989. Living with radiation. *National Geographic,* pp. 403–437.

Eisenbud, M. 1978. *Environment Technology and Health* (New York: University Press), p. 313.

Hendee, W. R. 1992. Estimation of radiation risks: BEIR V and its significance for medicine. *Journal of the American Medical Association* 268: 620–24.

Jablon, S., Z. Hrubec, J. D. Boice, and B. J. Stone. 1991. Cancer in populations living near nuclear facilities. *Journal of the American Medical Association* 265: 1403–1408.

Mays, C. W. 1988. Alpha-particle-induced cancer in humans. *Health Physics* 55: 637–52.

National Academy of Sciences Committee on Biological Effects of Ionizing Radiation (BEIR V). 1990. *Health Effects of Exposure to Low Levels of Ionizing Radiation.* Washington, D.C.

*Remmers, E. G. Spring 1989. Putting the risks into perspective:

Nuclear power. *Priorities,* p. 9.

Sagan, L. A. 1979. Medicine on the Midway. *Bulletin of the Medical Alumni Association* (Univ. of Chicago) 34.

Watkins, Admiral J. D. U.S. Secretary of Energy, in a speech on October 11, 1990 before the Heritage Associates.

*Whelan, E. M. 1978. *Preventing Cancer,* 1st ed. New York: W. W. Norton, p. 116.

Wing, S., C. M. Shy, J. L. Wood, et al. 1991. Mortality among workers at Oak Ridge National Laboratory—Evidence of radiation effects in following through 1984. *Journal of the American Medical Association* 265: 1397–1402.

Chapter 7: Sexual and Reproductive Patterns

American Cancer Society. October 1992. *Human Papillomaviruses.* Cancer Response System #2765.

Burns, M. K., C. D. Kennard, H. V. Dubin. 1991. Nodular cutaneous B-cell lymphoma of the scalp in the acquired immunodeficiency syndrome. *J. Am. Acad. Dermatol.* 25: 933–36.

Franco, E. L. 1991. Viral etiology of cervical cancer: A critique of the evidence. *Reviews of Infectious Diseases* 13: 1195–1206.

Gachupin-Garcia, A., P. A. Selwyn, N. S. Budner. 1992. Population-based study of malignancies and HIV infection among injecting drug users in a New York City methadone treatment program, 1985-1991. *AIDS* 6: 843–48.

Holladay, A. O., R. J. Siegel, and D. A. Schwartz. 1992. Cardiac malignant lymphoma in acquired immune deficiency syndrome. *Cancer* 70: 2203–2207.

Hulka, B. S. 1990. Hormone-replacement therapy and the risk of breast cancer. *CA: A Cancer Journal for Clinicians* 40: 289–96.

Larsen, P. M., M. Vetner, K. Nansen, and S. J. Fey, 1988. Future trends in cervical cancer. *Cancer Letters* 41: 123–37.

Molinari, J. A. 1991. Oral manifestations of HIV infection. *Journal of the Michigan Dental Association* 74: 38–43.

Pluda, J. M., S. Broder, and R. Yarchoan. 1992. Therapy of AIDS and AIDS-associated neoplasms. *Cancer Chemotherapy and Biological Response Modifiers Annual* 13. Elsevier Science Publishers B.V.

Skrabanek, P. 1988. Cervical cancer in nuns and prostitutes: A plea for scientific continence. *J. Clin. Epidemiol.* 41: 577–82.

Chapter 8: Medicines

Adler. E. H., and Weisstein, B. 1941. The clinical use of Stilbestrol. *Ohio State Med. Jour.* 37:945.

Bertling, M. Y., et al. 1950. DES in nausea and vomiting of pregnancy. *American Jour. of Obstet. and Gynec.* 59:461.

Blamey, R. W. 1969. Immunosuppression and cancer. *Lancet* 1:777.

Brody, H., and M. Cullen. 1957. Carcinoma of the breast seventeen years after mammography with Thorotrast. *Surgery* 42:600.

da Silva Horta, J., et al. 1965. Malignancy and other late effects following administration of Thorotrast. *Lancet* 2:201.

Dieckmann, W. J. 1953. Does the administration of DES during pregnancy have therapeutic value? *Amer. Jour. Obstet. Gynec.* 66:1062.

Fraumeni, J. F., and R. W. Miller. 1972. Drug induced cancer. *Jour. Natl. Cancer Inst.* 48:1267.

Gitman, L., and A. Koplowitz. 1950. Use of DES in complications of pregnancy. *New York State Med. Jour.* 50:2823.

Herbst, A., et al. 1971. Adenocarcinoma of the vagina: association of maternal Stilbestrol therapy with tumor appearance in young women. *New Eng. Jour. Med.* 284:878.

———. 1972. Vaginal and cervical abnormalities after exposure to Stilbestrol in utero. *Obstet. and Gynec.* 40:287.

————. 1974. Clear cell adenocarcinoma of the vagina and cervix in girls: Analysis of 170 registry cases. *Amer. Jour. of Obstet. Gynec.* 119:713.

————. 1975. Prenatal exposure to Stilbestrol: A prospective comparison of exposed female offspring with unexposed controls. *New Eng. Jour. Med.* 292:334.

Hoover, R., and J. F. Fraumeni. 1973. Risk of cancer in renal transplant recipients. *Lancet* 2:55.

————. 1975. Drugs. In *Persons at High Risk of Cancer,* ed. J F. Fraumeni. New York: Academic Press.

Hudgins, A. May 1943. Stilbestrol in obstetrics. *Medical Times.*

Jukes, T. H. Dec. 10, 1975. Estrogens in beef production. Unpublished.

Robinson, D., and L. B. Shettles. 1952. The use of DES in threatened abortion. *Amer. Jour. Obstet. and Gynec.* 63:1330.

Ryan, K. 1975. Cancer risk and estrogen use in the menopause. *New Eng. Jour. Med.* 293:1199.

Chapter 9: Occupation

Eide, I. 1990. A review of exposure conditions and possible health effects associated with aerosol and vapour from low-aromatic oil-based drilling fluids. *Ann. Occup. Hyg.* 34: 149–57.

Sankila, R. J., S. Karjalainen, H. M. Oksanen, et al. 1990. Relationship between occupation and lung cancer as analyzed by age and histologic type. *Cancer* 65: 1651–56.

Savitz, D. A., and J. Chen. 1990. Parental occupation and childhood cancer: Review of epidemiologic studies. *Environmental Health Perspectives* 88: 325–37.

Spinelli, J. J., P. R. Band, and R. P. Gallagher. 1990. Adjustment for confounding in occupational cancer epidemiology. *Recent Results Cancer Research* 120: 64–77.

Vineis, P., and L. Simonato. 1991. Proportion of lung and bladder cancers in males resulting from occupation: A systematic approach. *Archives of Environmental Health* 46: 6–15.

Chapter 10: Diet and Cancer

Adami, H.-O., et al. 1993. Report from the Working Group on Diet and Cancer. *Pharmacology and Toxicology* 72:S176–79.

*American Council on Science and Health. 1993. *Diet and Cancer.* New York.

*American Council on Science and Health. n.d. *Does Nature Know Best? Natural Carcinogens in American Food.* New York.

Ames, B. N. 1983. Dietary carcinogens and anticarcinogens: Oxygen radicals and degenerative diseases. *Science* 221: 1256–64.

Ausman, L. 1993. Fiber and colon cancer: Does the current evidence justify a preventive policy? *Nutrition Reviews* 51: 57–63.

Block, G. 1992. The data support a role for antioxidants in reducing cancer risk. *Nutrition Reviews* 50: 207–213.

———. 1992. Vitamin C status and cancer: Epidemiologic evidence of reduced risk. *Annals of the New York Academy of Sciences* 669: 280–90.

Block, G., B. Paterson, and A. Subar. 1992. Fruits, vegetables and cancer prevention: A review of the epidemiological evidence. *Nutrition and Cancer* 18: 1–29.

Byers, T., and G. Perry. 1992. Dietary carotenes, vitamin C, and vitamin E as protective antioxidants in human cancers. *Annual Review of Nutrition* 12: 139–59.

Etherton, G. M., and M. S. Kochar. 1993. Coffee: Factors and controversies. *Archives of Family Medicine* 2: 317–22.

Frudenheim, J. L., and S. Graham. 1992. Toward a dietary prevention of cancer. *Epidemiologic Reviews* 11: 229–35.

Howe, G., et al. 1991. The association between alcohol and breast cancer risk: Evidence from the combined analysis of sick dietary case-control studies. *International Journal of Cancer* 47: 707–710.

Howe, G. R. 1990. Dietary factors and risk of breast cancer: Combined analysis of 12 case-control studies. *Journal of the National Cancer Institute* 82: 561–69.

———. 1992. High-fat diets and breast cancer risk: The epidemiologic risk. *Journal of the American Medical Association* 268: 2080–81.

Kelsey, J. L., and M. D. Gammon. 1990. Epidemiology of breast cancer. *Epidemiologic Reviews* 12: 228–40.

Knekt, P., et al. 1991. Vitamin E and cancer prevention. *American Journal of Clinical Nutrition* 53: 283S–286S.

Kritchevsky, D. January/February 1993. Caloric restriction and experimental tumorigenesis. *Nutrition Today,* pp. 25–27.

Nomura, A. M. Y., and L. N. Kolonel. 1991. Prostate cancer: A current perspective. *American Journal of Epidemiology* 13: 200–227.

Roebuck, B. D. 1992. Dietary fat and the development of pancreatic cancer. *Lipids* 27: 804–806.

Rose, D. B., and Connolly. 1992. Dietary fat, fatty acids and prostate cancer. *Lipids* 27: 798–803.

Scheuplein, R. J. 1990. Perspectives on toxicological risk—an example: Food-borne carcinogenic risk. In *Progress in Predictive Toxicology,* ed. D. B. Clayson, et al. Elsevier Science Publishers B.V.

Trock, B., E. Lanza, and P. Greenwald. 1990. Dietary fiber, vegetables and colon cancer: Critical review and meta-analyses of the epidemiologic evidence. *Journal of the National Cancer Institute* 82: 650–61.

Ziegler, R. G. 1991. Vegetables, fruits and carotenoids and the risk of cancer. *American Journal of Clinical Nutrition* 53: 251S–259S.

Chapter 11: Exploding Myths about Purely Hypothetical Causes of Cancer

American Cancer Society. July 12, 1991. Cancer Response System #2681.

Bearsley, T. March 1991. Guessing game: The EPA tries to decide if there's harm from ELF. *Scientific American*, pp. 30–33.

Brown, H. D., and S. K. Chattopadhyay. 1988. Electromagnetic-field exposure and cancer. *Cancer Biochem Biophys* 9: 295–342.

Florig, H. K. 1992. *Science* 257: 468–92.

Gyuk, I. 1990. *Mitigation of Potential Health Hazards of Transmission Line Fields*. U.S. Department of Energy.

Kirkpatrick, D. March 8, 1993. Do cellular phones cause cancer? *Fortune* 127, pp. 26–31.

Morgan, M. G. 1989. *Electric and Magnetic Fields from 60 Hertz Electric Power: What Do We Know About Possible Health Risks?* Department of Engineering and Public Policy, Carnegie Mellon University.

National Cancer Institute. March 1990. *Questions and Answers: Collaborative Study of EMF Exposure and Childhood Leukemia*.

Sagan, L. A. 1992. Epidemiological and laboratory studies of power frequency electric and magnetic fields. *JAMA* 268: 625–29.

Salvatore, J. R., and A. B. Weitberg. 1989. Non-ionizing electromagnetic radiation and cancer—is there a relationship? *RI Med. J.* 72: 15–21.

Stevens, R. G., S. Davis, D. B. Thomas, et al. 1992. Electric power, pineal function and the risk of breast cancer. *FASEB J.* 6:853–60.

Stone, R. 1992. Polarized debate: EMFs and cancer. *Science* 258: 1724–25.

Theriault, G. 1990. Cancer risks due to exposure to electromagnetic fields. *Recent Results in Cancer Research* 120: 166–80.

Chapter 12: Screening for Early Detection of Cancer

*American Council on Science and Health. 1993. *Aspirin and Health: Impressive New Health Benefits of a Very Old Remedy.*

*American Council on Science and Health. 1986. *Cancer Screening: What You Can Do to Detect Cancer.*

*Coleman, R. L. Summer 1992. Cervical cancer: Causes and prevention. *Priorities.*

*Dittman, R. E. Winter 1993. Screening our children for cancer. *Priorities.*

Faivre, J., M. Wilpart, and M. C. Boutron. 1991. Primary prevention of large bowel cancer. *Recent Results in Cancer Research* 122: 85–99.

Jarvinen, J. H. 1988. Familial cancer. *Acta Oncologica* 27: 783–86.

Mettlin, C., G. Jones, H. Averette, S. B. Gusberg, and G. P. Murphy. 1993. Defining and updating the American Cancer Society guidelines for the cancer-related checkup: Prostate and endometrial cancers. *CA: A Cancer Journal for Clinicians* 43: 42–46.

Miller, B. A., E. J. Feuer, and B. F. Hankey. 1993. Recent incidence trends for breast cancer in women and the relevance of early detection: An update. *CA: A Cancer Journal for Clinicians* 43: 27–41.

*Whelan, E. M. October 1992. What they don't tell you about prostate cancer. *Across the Board.*

Wogan, G. N. 1992. Molecular epidemiology in cancer risk assessment and prevention: Recent progress and avenues for future research. *Environmental Health Perspectives* 9(S): 167–68.

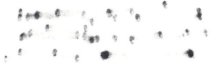

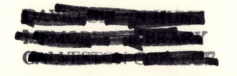

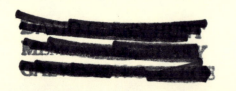